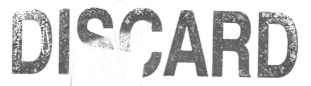
HEALERS ABROAD

Americans Responding to the Human Resource Crisis in HIV/AIDS

Committee on the Options for Overseas Placement of
U.S. Health Professionals

Board on Global Health

Fitzhugh Mullan, Claire Panosian, Patricia Cuff, *Editors*

INSTITUTE OF MEDICINE
OF THE NATIONAL ACADEMIES

THE NATIONAL ACADEMIES PRESS
Washington, D.C.
www.nap.edu

THE NATIONAL ACADEMIES PRESS 500 Fifth Street, N.W. Washington, DC 20001

NOTICE: The project that is the subject of this report was approved by the Governing Board of the National Research Council, whose members are drawn from the councils of the National Academy of Sciences, the National Academy of Engineering, and the Institute of Medicine. The members of the committee responsible for the report were chosen for their special competences and with regard for appropriate balance.

This study was supported by Contract No. SAQMPD04C1177 (STAT-6050) between the National Academy of Sciences and Office of the U.S. Global AIDS Coordinator at the U.S. Department of State. Any opinions, findings, conclusions, or recommendations expressed in this publication are those of the author(s) and do not necessarily reflect the view of the organizations or agencies that provided support for this project.

Library of Congress Cataloging-in-Publication Data

Institute of Medicine (U.S.). Committee on the Options for Overseas
   Placement of U.S. Health Professionals.
   Healers abroad : Americans responding to the human resource crisis in HIV/AIDS / Committee on the Options for Overseas Placement of U.S. Health Professionals, Board on Global Health ; Fitzhugh Mullan, Claire Panosian, Patricia Cuff, editors.
      p. ; cm.
   Includes bibliographical references.
   ISBN 0-309-09616-2 (pbk.)
   1. AIDS (Disease)—Government policy—United States. 2. Medical assistance, American.
3. World health.   I. Mullan, Fitzhugh. II. Panosian, Claire. III. Cuff, Patricia A. IV. Title.
   [DNLM: 1. HIV Infections—therapy. 2. Delivery of Health Care—organization & administration. 3. Health Manpower. 4. Health Personnel—education. 5. Health Planning. 6. International Cooperation.   WC 503.2 I589h 2005]
   RA643.8.I575 2005
   362.196′9792—dc22
                                          2005014301

Additional copies of this report are available from the National Academies Press, 500 Fifth Street, N.W., Lockbox 285, Washington, DC 20055; (800) 624-6242 or (202) 334-3313 (in the Washington metropolitan area); Internet, http://www.nap.edu.

For more information about the Institute of Medicine, visit the IOM home page at: **www.iom.edu.**

Suggested citation: Institute of Medicine. 2005. *Healers Abroad: Americans Responding to the Human Resource Crisis in HIV/AIDS.* Washington, DC: The National Academies Press.

Cover: "Community Embroidery" by the Paper Prayers Campaign and the Artist Proof Studio, 2001. The Community Embroidery was commissioned in South Africa by the inter-government committee on AIDS to show their commitment to preventing the spread of HIV/AIDS. It was implemented by the Paper Prayers Campaign, an outreach project of the Artist Proof Studio in Newtown. The embroidery was designed by a student of the Artist Proof Studio and embroidered by the Chivurika Embroidery group in Giyani, Limpopo Province, South Africa.

The serpent has been a symbol of long life, healing, and knowledge among almost all cultures and religions since the beginning of recorded history. The serpent adopted as a logotype by the Institute of Medicine is a relief carving from ancient Greece, now held by the Staatliche Museen in Berlin.

"Knowing is not enough; we must apply.
Willing is not enough; we must do."
—Goethe

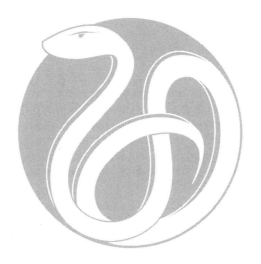

INSTITUTE OF MEDICINE
OF THE NATIONAL ACADEMIES

Adviser to the Nation to Improve Health

THE NATIONAL ACADEMIES
Advisers to the Nation on Science, Engineering, and Medicine

The **National Academy of Sciences** is a private, nonprofit, self-perpetuating society of distinguished scholars engaged in scientific and engineering research, dedicated to the furtherance of science and technology and to their use for the general welfare. Upon the authority of the charter granted to it by the Congress in 1863, the Academy has a mandate that requires it to advise the federal government on scientific and technical matters. Dr. Bruce M. Alberts is president of the National Academy of Sciences.

The **National Academy of Engineering** was established in 1964, under the charter of the National Academy of Sciences, as a parallel organization of outstanding engineers. It is autonomous in its administration and in the selection of its members, sharing with the National Academy of Sciences the responsibility for advising the federal government. The National Academy of Engineering also sponsors engineering programs aimed at meeting national needs, encourages education and research, and recognizes the superior achievements of engineers. Dr. Wm. A. Wulf is president of the National Academy of Engineering.

The **Institute of Medicine** was established in 1970 by the National Academy of Sciences to secure the services of eminent members of appropriate professions in the examination of policy matters pertaining to the health of the public. The Institute acts under the responsibility given to the National Academy of Sciences by its congressional charter to be an adviser to the federal government and, upon its own initiative, to identify issues of medical care, research, and education. Dr. Harvey V. Fineberg is president of the Institute of Medicine.

The **National Research Council** was organized by the National Academy of Sciences in 1916 to associate the broad community of science and technology with the Academy's purposes of furthering knowledge and advising the federal government. Functioning in accordance with general policies determined by the Academy, the Council has become the principal operating agency of both the National Academy of Sciences and the National Academy of Engineering in providing services to the government, the public, and the scientific and engineering communities. The Council is administered jointly by both Academies and the Institute of Medicine. Dr. Bruce M. Alberts and Dr. Wm. A. Wulf are chair and vice chair, respectively, of the National Research Council.

www.national-academies.org

COMMITTEE ON THE OPTIONS FOR OVERSEAS PLACEMENT OF U.S. HEALTH PROFESSIONALS

FITZHUGH MULLAN (*Chair*), *Health Affairs*/Project Hope and the Department of Prevention and Community Health, George Washington University School of Public Health and Health Services, Washington, DC

MICHELE BARRY, Office of International Health, Yale University School of Medicine, New Haven, CT

JANE Y. CARTER, African Medical and Research Foundation, Nairobi, Kenya

LINCOLN C. H. CHEN, Global Equity Initiative, Harvard University, Asia Center, Boston, MA

GARY GUNDERSON, Rollins School of Public Health, Emory University, Atlanta, GA

MALCOLM BARRY KISTNASAMY, Nelson R. Mandela School of Medicine, University of KwaZulu Natal, South Africa

RONALDO LIMA, International AIDS Vaccine Initiative, New York, NY

LESLIE D. MANCUSO, JHPIEGO Corporation at Johns Hopkins University, Baltimore, MD

WILLIAM MOORE, Clinical Professor of Medicine, Vanderbilt University, Nashville, TN

ANDRE-JACQUES NEUSY, Center for Global Health, New York University School of Medicine, New York, NY

JAMES B. PEAKE, Former U.S. Army Surgeon General and Project Hope Executive Vice President, Millwood, VA

CHRISTINA POLYAK, University of Maryland School of Medicine, Baltimore, MD

MARLA E. SALMON, Nell Hodgson Woodruff School of Nursing and Lillian Carter Center for International Nursing, Emory University, Atlanta, GA

ROBERT T. SCHOOLEY, Division of Infectious Diseases, University of California, San Diego

HARRISON C. SPENCER, Association of Schools of Public Health, Washington, DC

Liaisons and Study Consultants

THOMAS DENNY, Consultant
RICHARD GUERRANT, Board on Global Health Liaison
BJORG PALSDOTTIR, Consultant
CLAIRE PANOSIAN, Senior Consultant/Writer
KAI SPRATT, Consultant

Staff

PATRICK KELLEY, Board Director
PATRICIA CUFF, Program Officer
ALYSON SCHWABER, Research Associate/Assistant Editor
DIANNE STARE, Research Assistant
ALLISON BERGER, Senior Program Assistant

Staff

PATRICK KELLEY, Director
ALLISON BERGER, Senior Program Assistant
EILEEN CHOFFNES, Senior Program Officer
HEATHER COLVIN, Program Officer
PATRICIA CUFF, Program Officer
ALICIA GABLE, Senior Program Officer
HELLEN GELBAND, Senior Program Officer
AMY GIAMIS, Senior Program Assistant
STACEY KNOBLER, Senior Program Officer
KATHERINE OBERHOLTZER, Research Associate
MICHELE ORZA, Scholar/Study Director
ALYSON SCHWABER, Research Associate
LAURA SIVITZ, Research Associate
PENELOPE SMITH, Research Associate
DIANNE STARE, Research Assistant
KIMBERLY WEINGARTEN, Senior Program Assistant
JULIE WILTSHIRE, Financial Associate

Reviewers

This report has been reviewed in draft form by individuals chosen for their diverse perspectives and technical expertise, in accordance with procedures approved by the National Research Council's Report Review Committee. The purpose of this independent review is to provide candid and critical comments that will assist the institution in making its published report as sound as possible and to ensure that the report meets institutional standards for objectivity, evidence, and responsiveness to the study charge. The review comments and draft manuscript remain confidential to protect the integrity of the deliberative process. We wish to thank the following individuals for their review of this report:

J. Lyle Bootman, Arizona Health Sciences Center, University of Arizona, Tucson, Arizona

Larry Culpepper, Boston University Medical Center, Boston, Massachusetts

John Idoko, Jos University Teaching Hospital, Jos, Nigeria

Noddy Jinabhai, School of Family and Public Health, Nelson R. Mandela School of Medicine, University of KwaZulu-Natal, Durban, South Africa

Peter Okaalet, MAP International, Nairobi, Kenya

Jean W. Pape, Weill Medical College of Cornell University, New York

Susan C. Scrimshaw, University of Illinois, Chicago, Illinois

Deborah von Zinkernagel, Pangaea Global AIDS Foundation

Suwit Wibulpolprasert, Ministry of Public Health, Thailand

Although the reviewers listed above have provided many constructive comments and suggestions, they were not asked to endorse the conclusions or recommendations nor did they see the final draft of the report before its release. The review of this report was overseen by **Paul A. Volberding, M.D.**, Professor and Vice-Chair, Department of Medicine, University of California, San Francisco; and **Harold J. Fallon, M.D.**, Dean Emeritus, School of Medicine, University of Alabama at Birmingham. Appointed by the National Research Council and Institute of Medicine, they were responsible for making certain that an independent examination of this report was carried out in accordance with institutional procedures and that all review comments were carefully considered. Responsibility for the final content of this report rests entirely with the authoring committee and the institution.

Preface

Today, 14,000 people will contract HIV, and another 8,500 will die from AIDS. Malaria and tuberculosis (TB) will each claim roughly 3,000 more lives. These same cruel events will take place tomorrow and the next day and next week and next month. The death toll will only spiral upward as the HIV epidemic continues its global spread.

The terrible pandemic of HIV/AIDS has triggered an extraordinary response—a global counterattack mounted by international organizations, national governments, private philanthropies, pharmaceutical companies, churches, and individuals. The United Nations Global Fund, the World Health Organization's 3 × 5 Initiative, The World Bank, the Bill and Melinda Gates Foundation, national foreign aid programs, numerous faith-based groups, corporations, and nongovernmental organizations are committing funds, medications, and personnel to the battle against HIV/AIDS. The U.S. government joined the battle in earnest when Congress enacted President George W. Bush's Emergency Plan for AIDS Relief (PEPFAR) and earmarked $15 billion for the campaign. This broad range of global commitments has brought about a new era of possibility in preventing and treating HIV/AIDS and caring for those affected by the disease.

The campaign against HIV/AIDS has no precedent. Smallpox was defeated by a globally coordinated search-and-destroy strategy requiring only a single patient encounter to deliver the vaccine. In contrast, the strategy of directly observed therapy that lies at the core of modern TB treatment necessitates daily patient contact over much of the treatment course and therefore a far larger health workforce. Fighting HIV/AIDS will require the daily delivery of medications and the clinical management of patients *for the rest of their lives*. The sheer volume of health workers—and support systems—needed to wage this battle is well beyond anything before required of a public health campaign. The challenge is compounded by a chronic paucity of doctors, nurses, and other health personnel in many of the low-income countries targeted by PEPFAR where the epidemic is most fulminant. Sub-Saharan Africa, for instance, bears 25 percent of the world's overall burden of disease and 60 percent of the world's HIV/AIDS burden but has only 1.3 percent of the world's health workforce. There is one physician for every 360 people in the United States as compared with one for every 30,000 in Mozambique; one nurse exists for every 125 people in the United States but only one for every 5,000 in Uganda. There are 11 pharmacists in Rwanda.

Simply put, fighting HIV/AIDS in much of the world means building human health care capacity. No meaningful counterattack can occur without an adequate force of qualified health personnel to plan, implement, and sustain the campaign. In recognition of this fact, the PEPFAR legislation called for a pilot program to mobilize U.S. health professionals to work overseas in support of the plan's mission. The Office of the U.S. Global AIDS Coordinator at the Department of State, in turn, asked the Institute of Medicine to convene a committee to conduct a rapid study of options for such a program and report its recommendations. Motivated by the urgency of the global need and the historic opportunity to contribute to public health policy, the committee carried out its change with intensity, speed, and a sense of mission.

Healers Abroad is the product of that effort. Drawing on the extensive and varied experience of the committee members, testimony from health workers in the field, and the published literature on the global health workforce, the committee recommends programs in six key areas. Implementation of these recommendations would augment and accelerate the mobilization of U.S. health personnel to PEPFAR focus countries to help strengthen health care capacity and develop collaborative partnerships abroad. The committee also recommends that these programs be managed in a closely coordinated fashion as the Global Health Service. The resulting program would both symbolize the commitment of the people of the United States and catalyze the movement of U.S. health personnel overseas to help in the global counterattack on HIV/AIDS. It would be a program with a human face, combining the powerful tradition of people-to-people assistance with the best in contemporary health science and information technology. It would be a program of strategic humanitarianism, providing the support required by U.S. health professionals to assist people in need and to train counterpart health personnel abroad. The Global Health Service would help to stabilize societies at risk and demonstrate American compassion and civic spirit.

It is the committee's hope that this report will contribute to the success of PEPFAR and prove useful to others concerned with building a health workforce sufficient to meet the global HIV/AIDS challenge. It is our further hope that the report will be remembered as an early blueprint contributing to a new, enduring, and robust role for U.S. health professionals in improving global health.

Fitzhugh Mullan
Committee Chair

Acknowledgments

The committee recognizes the tremendous efforts of several individuals whose contributions invigorated discussions at its meetings and enhanced the quality of this report. For their expert advice, opinions, and willingness to assist, the committee thanks consultants Thomas Denny, Bjorg Palsdottir, and Kai Spratt, and its Board on Global Health liaison, Richard Guerrant. Special appreciation goes to writer and senior consultant Claire Panosian, whose skill in transforming ideas into words was instrumental in articulating the spirit of the committee's work. The committee also acknowledges with great thanks the testimony of Barbara Stilwell, Ummuro Adano, James Heiby, Gilbert Kombe, Antoine Augustin, Eric Krakauer, King Holmes, Col. Maureen Coleman, Gail Reed, Paul Dirdak, Ky Luu, Brian Palmer, Elise Frederick, Karen Hein, Ronald Campbell, Mike St. Louis, Thurma McCann Goldman, Don Weaver, Jack Hawkins, Nancy Kelly, Holly Burkhalter, Eric Friedman, Fred Valentine, Robert Einterz, Michael Scheld, Daniel Wikler, John Shippee, James Smith, Xingzhu Liu, Holly Ladd, and Rebecca Riccio. Additional thanks go to Stephen Moore, Annalisa Trama, Paul Moffat, Lydia Mungherera, and Chuka Anude for their written testimony from the field. Special recognition goes to Michael St. Louis, Estelle Quain, and Michele Moloney-Kitts for their extra effort and repeated attention to the ongoing provision of information and support for the study.

Joseph O'Neill, M.D., M.S., M.P.H., and Mark Dybul, M.D., of the Office of the U.S. Global AIDS Coordinator deserve particular recognition for generously supporting the vision that U.S. health professionals can make a difference in the fight against the global HIV/AIDS pandemic.

The committee would be remiss if it did not also acknowledge the hard work and dedication of the study staff from the Board on Global Health. Patrick Kelley, the director of the board, was an extremely valuable resource with his extensive knowledge of overseas placement of health professionals. We would also like to thank Patricia Cuff, study director, for her energy and commitment to ensuring that the report would be of the highest possible quality given the intense time pressure to complete the project. To Alyson Schwaber, research associate, the committee extends its utmost gratitude for her outstanding ability to examine critically and understand the research on overseas placement of health professionals. Dianne Stare did a remarkable job as research assistant, and Allison Berger performed equally well coordinating many of the study logistics. Final thanks are expressed to our editorial consultant Rona Briere and her steadfast assistant, Alisa Decatur.

Contents

APPENDIXES

Tables, Figures, and Boxes

TABLES

FIGURES

BOXES

Executive Summary

Human beings are the heart of health care. It is their labor and their intellect that translate science and technology into healing and hope. Just as oils and brushes without painters cannot create art, drugs and diagnostics without health workers cannot create health care. Nowhere is this more evident today than in the fight against global HIV/AIDS, the greatest health crisis of our time. As of this writing in 2005, close to 40 million people harbor HIV, 95 percent of whom live in resource-poor areas. Even before the pandemic hit, the health systems in these areas were weak and understaffed. Since the disease emerged, the dearth of health workers to treat and care for these HIV-infected individuals has reached crisis proportions.

The few health professionals practicing in many of the countries highly impacted by HIV/AIDS—workers often stressed, ill prepared, and scant in number—must now cope with a staggering new burden of disease while at the same time acquiring the knowledge, skills, and technology to deliver lifelong antiretroviral drug regimens, HIV/AIDS clinical and palliative care, and prevention services. Arguably, their task represents the most profound challenge in the scaling up of health care the world has ever known. They cannot accomplish this task alone.

In this context, this report explores potential strategies for mobilizing U.S. health personnel and technical experts to assist in the battle against HIV/AIDS in 15 African, Caribbean, and Southeast Asian countries highly affected by the disease. Commissioned by the U.S. Department of State as part of a historic global health initiative—the President's Emergency Plan for AIDS Relief (PEPFAR)—the report presents the results of a study conducted by the Institute of Medicine's Committee on the Options for Overseas Placement of U.S. Health Professionals. In carrying out this study, the committee:

- Reviewed available data sources to project the optimum size and composition of a U.S. global health professions service program to augment, train, and collaborate with the public health and clinical professionals residing in the host countries
- Assessed the relative strengths and weaknesses of existing and potential organizational models for such a program that could rapidly be activated or adapted to recruit, train, and place program participants
- Articulated principles that can be applied in evaluating the advantages and disadvantages of those models
- Examined other contextual issues bearing on the successful implementation of a U.S. global health professions service program

In this report, the committee recommends a set of interconnected workforce enhancement programs that would meet the need to augment the health professional currently waging the fight against HIV/AIDS and other global diseases. The committee believes that, given adequate resources, talent, and political will, these programs would make an enormous contribution to the eventual control of these terrible afflictions.

HUMAN RESOURCES FOR HEALTH

The health workforce in low-income countries has suffered from years of national and international neglect. Indeed, the dearth of qualified health care professionals represents the single greatest obstacle to meeting health care needs in most low-income countries (Narasimhan et al., 2004). The World Health Organization's (WHO) Commission on Macroeconomics and Health recently advocated a greatly increased investment in health, reaching a per capita expenditure of $34 per year in low-income countries. At the same time, WHO stated that the main barrier to implementing this increased investment is not funding, but the capacity of the health sector itself to absorb the increased flow (Habte et al., 2004). As new resources continue to be mobilized to fight HIV/AIDS, tuberculosis, malaria, and other diseases, it is most unfortunate that an insufficient workforce is impeding the success of these investments. External grants and funding to address global HIV/AIDS, estimated at $5 billion in 2003, could reach $20 billion by 2007 (UNAIDS, 2004). At present, however, there is simply too little human capacity in many developing countries to absorb, apply, and make efficient use of these new funds and critical health initiatives.

What underlies the health workforce crisis? In many countries, including those with a high prevalence of HIV/AIDS, the inability to recruit and retain an effective, well-motivated, appropriately skilled health workforce stems not only from HIV/AIDS itself, but from other problems as well, including low pay and morale, poor work conditions, and weak management. Some workers experience a combination of understaffed workplaces, low compensation, and civil service or public expenditure reforms that prevent recruitment of new staff. In recent years, these factors have fueled a trend for some health professionals to move from the public to the private sector, to migrate internationally in pursuit of more favorable opportunities, or to abandon their profession altogether.

The problem of insufficient human resources for health care is most acute in sub-Saharan Africa, which bears 25 percent of the world's overall burden of disease but houses only 1.3 percent of the world's health workforce. Currently, an estimated 750,000 health workers serve the 682 million people of sub-Saharan Africa. By comparison, the ratio of health care workers to population is 10 to 15 times higher in the countries of the Organization for Economic Cooperation and Development (HLF, 2004).

COMPREHENSIVE CARE FOR HIV/AIDS IN DEVELOPING COUNTRIES

The prevention, care, and treatment of HIV/AIDS in developing countries will require unprecedented health systems and human resources to deliver medications and oversee patients *for the rest of their lives*. Ideally, a comprehensive approach to HIV/AIDS includes a range of components, including the following:

- Community and national treatment, care, and prevention guidelines
- Education and awareness programs
- Programs to address stigma and discrimination
- Voluntary counseling and testing with informed consent in health facilities, along with services targeting vulnerable and difficult-to-reach populations
- Prevention of mother-to-child transmission
- Prevention and treatment of opportunistic and sexually transmitted infections
- Antiretroviral therapy and monitoring, including essential laboratory and clinical backup and drug management systems
- Embedded operations research programs designed to elucidate the most effective approaches to HIV/AIDS care and delivery in resource-limited settings
- Adherence support
- Social protection, nutrition, and welfare and psychosocial services

- Palliative and home-based care
- Bereavement support

In reality, however, models of health care delivery for HIV/AIDS must first reflect the capacities of host countries. For example, antiretroviral therapy should be initiated only if certain minimum conditions are met, including community preparedness, counseling and testing with informed consent, training of personnel for provision of antiretroviral drugs and follow-up, clinical and laboratory monitoring, reliable drug delivery systems, and education to maximize adherence. Should these conditions not be met, one of the gravest outcomes could be the emergence and wide-scale spread of resistance to antiretroviral drugs, an occurrence that would ultimately jeopardize the future treatment of all infected persons and populations around the world. Preventing such a catastrophe will require appropriate training, support, accreditation, and quality control of providers in both the public and private sectors during the scale-up of antiretroviral therapy (WHO, 2003a).

Experience with pilot programs has revealed several ways to integrate prevention and care efforts through various clinical entry points, including voluntary counseling and testing, sexual and reproductive health services, and other health services.

Voluntary Counseling and Testing

Voluntary counseling and testing with informed consent is the key point at which people learn their HIV status and are offered care services, as well as behavioral and preventive advice. Studies have shown that voluntary counseling and testing consistently increases safe-sex behaviors (CDC, 2000; Spielberg et al., 2003; The Voluntary HIV-1 Counseling and Testing Efficacy Study Group, 2000; Weinhardt et al., 1999). Until recently, however, access to such services in countries most severely affected by HIV/AIDS has been limited. As a result, there are few developing countries in which more than 10 percent of the adult population has been tested (Fylkesnes and Siziya, 2004). Increased provision of voluntary counseling and testing services in developing countries—reaching geographically remote areas as well as community clinics and networks—must parallel the scale-up of other HIV-related efforts. Otherwise, limited availability of these services could prove to be an impediment to expanded treatment and care (Heiby, 2004).

Maternal–Child Services

Antenatal services provide access to programs designed to prevent mother-to-child transmission of HIV and to allow HIV-infected women to receive treatment and care during and after pregnancy, as well as advice for future pregnancies (WHO, 2003b). As part of worldwide efforts to expand access to such services and to antiretroviral therapy, routine testing of pregnant women (with the right to refuse) is recommended in the 2004 joint United Nations/WHO policy statement on HIV testing (UNAIDS Global Reference Group on HIV/AIDS and Human Rights, 2004). Without intervention, 35 to 40 percent of HIV-positive women transmit the infection to their infants; with drug prophylaxis and formula feeding, transmission is reduced to 5 to 10 percent, while with combination antiretroviral therapy, transmission falls below 1 percent (Nolan et al., 2002).

Caregiving and Palliation

Despite new global initiatives, many medically eligible patients in developing countries will not receive antiretroviral therapy over the next few years. Caregiving and palliative measures—generally defined as pain and symptom management, advance care planning, prioritization of life goals, and support for individuals and families throughout the course of disease—will be essential elements of all comprehensive HIV/AIDS programs. The provision of such services is a pressing need in Asia (Coughlan, 2003) as well as in Africa (Ramsay, 2003). One survey of 48 palliative care services for patients with AIDS in Africa found that 94 percent had faced obstacles, especially a lack of trained providers, stigma, and government restrictions on access to such palliative treatments as oral morphine. Yet medically treating and controlling pain and other symptoms in the terminal phases of AIDS allows many patients to stay in their homes without the cost or disruption of transferring them to hospitals (Harding et al., 2003).

THE PRESIDENT'S EMERGENCY PLAN FOR AIDS RELIEF

During his State of the Union address on January 28, 2003, President George W. Bush announced the $15 billion PEPFAR initiative, with the following 5-year goals: (1) providing antiretroviral therapy for 2 million people; (2) preventing 7 million new HIV infections; and (3) providing care to 10 million people infected with or affected by HIV/AIDS, including orphans and vulnerable children. In May 2003, the U.S. Congress passed authorizing legislation (United States Leadership against HIV/AIDS, Tuberculosis, and Malaria Act of 2003) for the plan. Legislative provisions recommended the following targeted distribution of funds: treatment (55 percent), prevention (20 percent), palliative care (15 percent), and care of orphans and vulnerable persons (10 percent). This unprecedented global health initiative placed the United States at the forefront of international efforts targeting HIV/AIDS. Today PEPFAR accounts for more than 50 percent of annual global funding.

PEPFAR now encompasses HIV/AIDS activities in more than 100 countries, but is focused on the development of comprehensive and integrated prevention, care, and treatment programs in 15 countries: Botswana, Cote d'Ivoire, Ethiopia, Guyana, Haiti, Kenya, Mozambique, Namibia, Nigeria, Rwanda, South Africa, Tanzania, Uganda, Zambia, and Vietnam. The original 14 countries in Africa and the Caribbean represent 50 percent of the world's HIV/AIDS burden. Vietnam was added to the list in July 2004 as a result of its projected eight-fold rise in HIV infections from 2002 to 2010 (Office of National AIDS Policy, 2004).

RECOMMENDATIONS

To meet the needs outlined above, the committee proposes the creation of a Global Health Service (GHS), a new national initiative encompassing six interconnected programs designed to mobilize, prepare, send, manage, and compensate U.S. health professionals for service in the 15 PEPFAR focus countries. The mission of the GHS is to be flexible and responsive to the needs for human resources for health identified by those countries whose citizens are most affected by the HIV/AIDS pandemic and other global scourges; to provide expertise in the form of clinicians, technical advisers, trainers, and mentors; and to establish enduring relationships among global colleagues. The following guiding principles frame the GHS effort as envisioned by the committee:

- Country responsiveness
- Interdisciplinary, cross-cutting approaches
- Training for self-sufficiency
- Nondepletion of the local health care workforce
- Multiplier effect
- Sustained involvement and ownership

The committee's first two recommendations address the creation of the GHS and the overall management of its six component programs. The six recommendations that follow deal in turn with each of those programs.

Recommendation 1: *Create a U.S. Global Health Service.* The committee discussed the importance of establishing a clear identity for programs designed to mobilize health personnel for service in combating HIV/AIDS in highly impacted countries. A well recognized identity—a brand—was felt to be essential to the creation of mission and the promotion of volunteerism. **Therefore the committee recommends the establishment of a U.S. Global Health Service to serve as the umbrella organization for the initiatives and programs to be proposed in this report.**

Recommendation 1a: *Mobilize providers and capacity developers.* The committee believes that a wide variety of health professionals and other key technical and management personnel will be essential for achieving the PEPFAR goals of treating 2 million HIV-infected people, preventing 7 million new HIV infections, and caring for 10 million HIV-affected individuals and vulnerable children (the 2-7-10 PEPFAR goals), as well as for building the long-term capacity necessary to control HIV/AIDS, tuberculosis, and malaria. Therefore, the committee recommends that the programs of the U.S. Global Health Service initially focus on the mobilization of clinicians, technicians, and management personnel in direct response to specified in-country needs to achieve PEPFAR goals. In view of the lack of human resources for health in PEPFAR focus countries and many other developing countries, education, training, and development of new, effective configurations of health care delivery in resource-poor settings will take high priority among the U.S. Global Health Service's activities.

As envisioned by the committee, the GHS encompasses a suite of programs under a single banner. The committee believes the parent program should be housed within the U.S. government, although certain activities and functions could be contracted to experienced nongovernmental organizations. A government-based program would enhance the international credibility, transparency, and clarity of purpose of the GHS; position it closer to the federal appropriations process; and sustain its close relationship to PEPFAR. In addition, a single management structure would serve as a focal point for legislation, budget, and administration while allowing the parent office to maximize efficiency and streamline operations. At the same time, however, the use of private-sector contracts and public–private partnerships is crucial to foster creative solutions, to supplement financing, and to enhance administrative flexibility. While a variety of programs to mobilize U.S. health professionals for service abroad already exist, none embodies the scope and values of the proposed GHS.

Recommendation 2: *Manage the programs of the U.S. Global Health Service in a unitary fashion.* The committee recommends that the programs of the U.S. Global Health Service be managed in a unitary fashion to provide maximum synergy, coordination, and clarity of purpose. Fiscal, administrative, and management matters should be handled by the single organizational entity that would be dedicated to the mission of mobilizing U.S. personnel to work in PEPFAR focus countries. Finally, in order for the U.S. Global Health Service to relate closely to PEPFAR and to participate in the annual federal budget process, the committee recommends that the U.S. Global Health Service should be a program of the federal government. In order to be successful, the U.S. Global Health Service needs to collaborate with the private sector, nongovernmental organizations, and public–private matching programs.

Public input to the management of such a high-visibility global program is important for maintaining a balanced view. The committee believes that the best mechanism to this end would be an external advisory committee. Recognizing the fundamental importance of involving partners in the development and ongoing operation of the GHS, the committee believes further that the members of the advisory committee should include colleagues from the PEPFAR focus countries and nongovernmental organizations, as well as other key collaborators from the United States and abroad.

Recommendation 2a: *Establish an advisory committee for the Global Health Service that includes international members.* The committee recognizes the fundamental importance of involving partners in the development and ongoing operation of the U.S. Global Health Service. These partners would include colleagues from nongovernmental organizations, PEPFAR countries, and other key collaborators from the Uniyed States and abroad. **The committee recommends the creation of a policy-level advisory committee with international colleagues and a commitment to the strategic engagement of public and private partners in the planning, operation, and evaluation of the U.S. Global Health Service.**

As noted above, the GHS envisioned by the committee encompasses six interconnected programs. The committee believes this package of programs would significantly augment human resource capacity in support of the PEPFAR goals outlined earlier. The six programs are as follows:

- Global Health Service Corps
- Health Workforce Needs Assessment
- Fellowship Program
- Loan Repayment Program
- Twinning Program
- Clearinghouse

Global Health Service Corps

The lack of skilled and trained health professionals is one of the principal barriers to the rapid scale-up of HIV/AIDS prevention and treatment programs in the PEPFAR focus countries (Adano et al., 2004; Wyss, 2004a, b). A range of skills is needed, particularly at the level of key clinical, managerial, and technical leadership positions essential to developing the infrastructure of HIV/AIDS treatment systems (WHO, 2002). Because of the specialized nature of these positions and the long-term requirements of the work, volunteer health professionals and those with short-term availability will be of limited utility in addressing core country-level needs. It would be the role of the Global Health Service Corps, working with public health leaders in the PEPFAR focus countries, to provide specialized health personnel for extended assignments to fill these positions and accelerate program scale-up. These highly skilled professionals would be full-salaried employees working in the 15 focus countries for extended periods, yet the cost of their salary and benefits is estimated roughly at only 1 percent of the total PEPFAR budget.

Recommendation 3: *Establish a U.S. Global Health Service Corps to send key health personnel to PEPFAR countries on a full-time/long-term basis.* **The committee recommends the establishment of a full-salaried/long-term U.S. Global Health Service Corps for the recruitment, placement, and support of U.S. health, technical, and management professionals in PEPFAR countries. Because of the critical and highly visible nature of this Corps and the necessity for it to coordinate closely with PEPFAR, the committee further recommends that it be established and administered as a program of the federal government.** U.S. Global Health Service Corps professionals should be selected and deployed based on the prioritized needs identified by ministries of health in conjunction with in-country PEPFAR teams. Assignments will be made for a minimum of 2 years with placements in areas and programs where Corps members' presence would have maximum impact on enhancing the human capacity to prevent and treat HIV/AIDS. The committee proposes an initial deployment of 150 U.S. Global Health Service Corps professionals in the 15 PEPFAR countries based on needs assessment, placement development, and the availability of professionals with the required skills.

Health Workforce Needs Assessment

The GHS would be responsible for sending health and other professionals from the United States to countries with substantiated needs for specific forms of assistance. Conducting an assessment of health workforce needs is therefore an essential early step (MSH, 2004). Currently, the PEPFAR countries vary in the ways they collect and analyze data on their human resource capacity for health care. Lack of consistency also characterizes the monitoring of health workforce development strategies in these countries (Diallo et al., 2003). Although all of the focus countries have strategic plans through the U.S. Agency for International Development, these plans were not designed to address human resource issues and are therefore not useful for the purpose. Country Plans drafted by U.S. government teams in each PEPFAR country were not available for review as of this writing.

Recommendation 4: *Undertake a uniform health workforce needs assessment.* The committee recommends that the PEPFAR country teams, in collaboration with ministries of health, initiate assessments of in-country requirements for health personnel to achieve PEPFAR goals. These assessments should form the basis for national human resources for health plans. These assessments would also generate a valuable baseline inventory for all mobilization programs and subsequent evaluation activities. The data from all countries should be collected in a standardized fashion, updated regularly, and maintained in the electronic database of the U.S. Global Health Service Clearinghouse "Opportunity Bank," available to professionals interested in service in PEPFAR countries. Timely and accurate information on workforce needs will be essential to maximize the impact of programs designed to mobilize health personnel to achieve PEPFAR goals. Current national needs assessments are irregular, nonstandardized, and not available at any single site. Local placement strategies and global recruitment efforts would be greatly strengthened by a regularized needs assessment and dissemination initiative.

Fellowship Program

The GHS Fellowship Program would provide incentives to encourage qualified health personnel who wish to work abroad to serve within the framework of the PEPFAR mission. The structure of the proposed fellowship program would engage professionals by reducing financial and logistical barriers, while also focusing their activities to align with the PEPFAR goals. Much like the prestigious Fulbright awards, the GHS Fellowships would confer honor and professional recognition on their recipients.

Recommendation 5: *Create a U.S. Global Health Service Fellowship Program.* The committee recommends the creation of a U.S. Global Health Service Fellowship Program that would provide professional recognition and a $35,000 award to qualified U.S. personnel to enable commitment to programs of service in PEPFAR countries. This competitive program would fund a prestigious award to individuals willing to make medium-term commitments of 1 year or longer to provide health care, training, and technical assistance in countries in need. It would provide career-long recognition as well as immediate financial assistance.

Loan Repayment Program

Given the growing levels of educational debt incurred by today's health professionals, loan repayment is a benefit that can reduce barriers to service. In the academic year 1996–97, medical students borrowed more than $1.11 billion, and fully 83.2 percent of the 1997 graduating class had incurred educational debt (Beran and Lawson, 1998). In 2003–04, tuition and fees at public medical schools averaged $16,153 and at private schools reached a staggering $32,588 (Jolly, 2004). This financial burden could potentially leave a young medical professional with a debt ranging from $140,000 to $255,000, making the concept of exchanging debt for service highly appealing (Morrison, 2005).

Recommendation 6: *Establish a U.S. Global Health Service Loan Repayment Program.* **The committee recommends the establishment of a U.S. Global Health Service Loan Repayment Program for clinical, managerial, and technical professionals prepared to serve for designated periods in PEPFAR focus countries. This program would provide $25,000 toward scholastic debt reduction for each year of service in PEPFAR focus countries.** Clinical, managerial, and technical professionals graduate from training programs today with substantial debts that limit their ability to consider voluntary or less remunerative work. A loan repayment program would expand the pool of professionals who could consider service abroad and make many more skilled individuals available to address PEPFAR goals.

Twinning Program

The establishment of partnerships between U.S. health professionals and local organizations such as hospitals, universities, nongovernmental organizations, and public health agencies—often referred to as twinning programs—offers a number of key advantages. Having such an existing structure can strengthen the host country workforce by allowing the rapid deployment of foreign health professionals to fill personnel voids, to provide relevant training together with colleagues in their host's home environment, and to train trainers who can facilitate expanded knowledge in specific areas such as HIV care and prevention (ICAD and CI, 2002). U.S. professionals could also temporarily substitute for local staff while the latter traveled off site for much-needed training. The ability offered by such programs to quickly mobilize U.S. personnel would be critical to short-staffed institutions in the PEPFAR focus countries.

Recommendation 7: *Promote twinning as a mechanism to mobilize health personnel.* The committee recommends long-term, targeted funding for innovative, institutional partnerships that would mobilize U.S. health personnel to work in PEPFAR countries. Often called "twinning," these bidirectional partnerships (which encompass counterpart organizations ranging from hospitals and universities to nongovernmental organizations and public health agencies) develop institutional capacities and create a sustainable relationship between the partners that extends beyond the life of the defined project. It is a bilateral arrangement that can develop collaboration in many areas but stands to be a particularly helpful instrument to augment teaching, training, and service capacities in combating HIV/AIDS. Twinning should be supported between a variety of U.S. and PEPFAR country-based institutions that are most relevant to meeting PEPFAR targets and harmonizing with PEPFAR country operating plans, especially public-sector health agencies. Twinning is a mechanism that can move skilled personnel from a sending organization to a host organization to provide support, training, and technical assistance. It provides a ready-made structure in host countries for U.S. health professionals to engage with maximum speed and effectiveness.

Clearinghouse

Many organizations currently send health professionals to work in the PEPFAR focus countries. Given their experience, these groups are well poised to assist in HIV/AIDS treatment, prevention, and care, thus helping to achieve the PEPFAR goals. A virtual network of such organizations could provide and receive relevant information and regularly reach thousands of volunteers.

Recommendation 8: *Develop a U.S. Global Health Service Clearinghouse.* There are many organizations currently mobilizing health personnel to work in PEPFAR countries. These organizations could be powerful allies in meeting PEPFAR goals. Therefore the committee recommends a multifaceted Clearinghouse for the U.S. Global Health Service that would facilitate information exchange, enhance access to program data, and provide opportunity information for interested health professionals.

The proposed Clearinghouse would include the following:

- **Program Resource Directory and Networks**—a searchable, web-based directory that would provide screened, reliable links enabling interested volunteers to view sending organizations' websites, thus facilitating organizational recruitment.
- **Opportunity Bank**—a job bank of available host-country positions that would be a valuable tool for U.S. professionals wishing to work in the PEPFAR focus countries as a volunteer or a paid employee.
- **Cultural and Strategic Issues Reference Site**—a virtual warehouse of information pertinent to all health professionals planning to work in the PEPFAR focus countries, including those seeking a GHS Fellowship, loan repayment, or assignments to the GHS Corps.
- **Country Credentials and Travel Guidelines Repository**—a compendium of updated virtual information designed to assist prospective volunteers in applying for work in the global arena.

LOOKING AHEAD

The committee concluded its work by considering various approaches holding promise for enhancing and sustaining the global health workforce in both low- and high-resource countries into the future.

Development of Long-Term Health Workforce Capacity

The GHS is envisioned as a strategic and humanitarian intervention in settings that currently lack sufficient human resources for health to mount a counterattack on HIV/AIDS. The six programs of the GHS are not intended to produce a permanent workforce or to substitute for the development of health personnel capacity in the PEPFAR nations. The long-term sustainability of the program must be a priority for both the PEPFAR countries and the United States. Over time, all the PEPFAR countries will have to develop sufficiently capable and sustainable workforces to continue HIV/AIDS prevention and treatment programs into the foreseeable future. There is a strong rationale for U.S. health professionals, as well as other foreign workers, to help establish self-sufficiency in these countries through training, skill development, partnership, and other forms of human resource support.

The committee believes that national capacity development in each PEPFAR focus country should entail the following steps:

1. Each country should undertake a health workforce needs assessment as part of or a complement to its overall national plan.

2. National education and training should be accelerated to develop the human resources needed to address the HIV/AIDS epidemic and meet primary health care needs.

3. The work environment for health professionals should ensure staff retention and encourage employees to maintain an acceptable level of job performance.

4. The "brain drain" should be stopped by dampening demand in richer countries that continue to recruit skilled health workers.

5. Where necessary, priority programs and health systems should be harmonized to avoid fragmentation, duplication, and waste.

Although the development of long-term health professional capacity must be a priority for host countries, the United States can take significant actions to assist in the effort. Foremost among these is investing in the development of health workforce capacity. Medical and nursing schools need to be built and staffed. Midlevel provider programs that offer continuing education and advanced training need to be promoted and funded. Community and village health workers need to be trained by the thousands and equipped with standardized basic skills for HIV/AIDS work.

At the same time, the United States has a key role to play in creating stability in the health sector of developing countries by ending the brain drain of physicians, nurses, and other skilled health personnel. This out-migration is triggered by the failure of the United States and other developed nations to educate sufficient health professionals to meet their domestic needs (Stilwell et al., 2004). The resultant exodus of scarce human resources is a prominent barrier to building in the health workforce needed in the PEPFAR focus countries to meet the increased demands of HIV/AIDS treatment and prevention.

Creative Partnerships

Increasingly employed in comprehensive development frameworks, public–private partnerships have featured prominently in international health in recent years. In 2003, 91 international arrangements in the health sector qualified as public–private partnerships; 76 of these were dedicated to the control of HIV/AIDS or other infectious diseases. Notable examples include partnerships orchestrated principally by large multinational companies, as well as those initiated by nongovernmental organizations working with corporations. Individual governments have also formed partnerships with for-profit private entities or nongovernmental organizations with particular technical or outreach strengths. A variety of creative public–private partnerships focused on the health workforce mission of PEPFAR can be envisioned. The committee believes that alliances between the GHS and the private sector in particular should be supported and encouraged.

E-Health

E-health is defined as the use of technology to exchange actionable information to facilitate the delivery of health services. E-health allows health professionals to overcome barriers of time and distance, bringing expertise, education, and training to remote locations and providing services that poor, isolated communities would otherwise lack. An example is the use of personal digital assistants for the management of antiretroviral therapy, patient record keeping, patient tracking, data collection, and knowledge building. Such e-health applications could support the scale-up of HIV/AIDS care and treatment in PEPFAR focus countries by:

- Enabling health care workers to increase their efficiency and effectiveness
- Providing the local health care establishment with immediate access to experts and expert centers in the United States and elsewhere
- Offering individual support to overseas professionals to enable and encourage longer deployments

Global Health Education in the United States

Global health education is more than the study of diseases of the developing world; it involves a matrix of many converging factors—economic, cultural, historical, political, and environmental—that influence health and disease worldwide. Interest in global health among U.S. medical students and postgraduate residents is currently at a high level; in 2003, more than 20 percent of students graduating from U.S. medical schools spent time abroad, compared with just 6 percent in 1984 (AAMC, 1984, 2003). This level of interest suggests that a sizable pool of U.S. health professionals is open to overseas work opportunities linked to global service. To meet the educational needs of these students and the national interests of the United States, the committee supports upgraded, multidisciplinary global health curricula and appropriate professional consortia within both health professional schools and other educational settings.

THE CHOICE TO ACT

This report proposes a set of measures with the potential to augment and accelerate the mobilization of U.S. health professionals for the battle against HIV/AIDS. Each of these measures represents an option that could be adopted either by using the current PEPFAR authority or by initiating new legislative or administrative action. The idea of a Global Health Service, however, goes far beyond its individual elements. HIV is global, relentless, and highly mutable—a truly terrifying adversary. The counterattack against HIV/AIDS must be equally bold and inventive, marshaling science, financial resources, and personal commitment. The GHS is proposed as an instrument of such a counterattack, an organization that would appeal to the heads and hearts of U.S. health professionals and engage them in growing numbers to join the campaign against the global scourge of HIV/AIDS.

REFERENCES

AAMC (Association of American Medical Colleges). 1984. *Medical School Graduation Questionnaire All Schools Report*. Washington, DC: AAMC.

AAMC. 2003. *Medical School Graduation Questionnaire All Schools Report*. Washington, DC: AAMC.

Adano U, O'Neil M, Decima E, Kiarie W. 2004. *Rapid Assessment of the Human Resource Implications of Scaling Up HIV/AIDS Services in Uganda Progress Report 1 & 2*. Management and Leadership Development Project/USAID. Boston, MA: Management Sciences for Health.

Beran RL, Lawson GE. 1998. Medical student financial assistance, 1996–1997. *Journal of the American Medical Association* 280:819–820.

CDC (Centers for Disease Control and Prevention). 2000. Adoption of protective behaviors among persons with recent HIV infection and diagnosis—Alabama, New Jersey, and Tennessee, 1997–1998. *Morbidity and Mortality Weekly Report* 49(23):512–515.

Coughlan M. 2003. Pain and palliative care for people living with HIV/AIDS in Asia. *Journal of Pain & Palliative Care Pharmacotherapy* 17(3-4):91–104; discussion 105–106.

Diallo K, Zurn P, Gupta N, Dal Poz M. 2003. Monitoring and evaluation of human resources for health: An international perspective. *Human Resources for Health* 1(3).

Fylkesnes K, Siziya S. 2004. A randomized trial on acceptability of voluntary HIV counselling and testing. *Tropical Medicine and International Health* 9(5):566–572.

Habte D, Dussault G, Dovlo D. 2004. Challenges confronting the health workforce in sub-Saharan Africa. *World Hospitals & Health Services* 40(2):23–26, 40–41.

Harding R, Stewart K, Marconi K, O'Neill JF, Higginson IJ. 2003. Current HIV/AIDS end-of-life care in sub-Saharan Africa: A survey of models, services, challenges and priorities. *Biomed Central Public Health* 3(1):33.

Heiby J. 2004. (December 1). *Quality of Care and Human Resources in HIV Healthcare Programs*. Presentation at the December 1, 2004, Workshop of the IOM Committee on Options for the Overseas Placement of U.S. Health Professionals, Washington, DC.

HLF (High Level Forum on the Health Millennium Development Goals). 2004. *Addressing Africa's Health Workforce Crisis: An Avenue for Action*. Abuja, Nigeria: World Bank and WHO.

ICAD and CI (Inter-agency Coalition on AIDS and Development and Communication Initiative). 2002. *Twinning Against AIDS*. Quebec, Canada: Canadian International Development Agency. [Online]. Available: http://www.comminit.com/pdf/twinning_against_AIDS_Final_Report.pdf [accessed March 11, 2005].

Jolly P. 2004. *Medical School Tuition and Young Physician Indebtedness.* Washington, DC: AAMC.

Morrison G. 2005. Mortgaging our future: The cost of medical education. *New England Journal of Medicine* 352(2):117–119.

MSH (Management Sciences for Health). 2004. Tackling the crisis in human capacity development for health services. *The Manager* 13(2):1–20.

Narasimhan V, Brown H, Pablos-Mendez A, Adams O, Dussault G, Elzinga G, Nordstrom A, Habte D, Jacobs M, Solimano G, Sewankambo N, Wibulpolprasert S, Evans T, Chen L. 2004. Responding to the global human resources crisis. *Lancet* 363(9419):1469–1472.

Nolan ML, Greenberg AE, Fowler MG. 2002. A review of clinical trials to prevent mother-to-child HIV-1 transmission in Africa and inform rational intervention strategies. [Review] [51 refs]. *AIDS* 16(15):1991–1999.

Office of National AIDS Policy. 2004. *Fact Sheet: Extending and Improving the Lives of Those Living with HIV/AIDS.* [Online]. Available: http://www.whitehouse.gov/news/releases/2004/06/20040623-1.html [accessed March 1, 2005].

Ramsay S. 2003. Leading the way in African home-based palliative care. Free oral morphine has allowed expansion of model home-based palliative care in Uganda. *Lancet* 362(9398):1812–1813.

Spielberg F, Camp S, Ramachandra E. 2003 (July 27–30). *HIV Home Self-testing: Can It Work? (Abstract M1-A0101).* Presented at the July 27–30, 2003, National HIV Prevention Conference, Atlanta, GA.

Stilwell B, Diallo K, Zurn P, Vujicic M, Adams O, Dal Poz M. 2004. Migration of health care workers from developing countries: Strategic approaches to its management. *Bulletin of the World Health Organization* 82(8):559–636.

The Voluntary HIV-1 Counseling and Testing Efficacy Study Group. 2000. Efficacy of voluntary HIV-1 counseling and testing in individuals and couples in Kenya, Tanzania, and Trinidad: A randomized trial. *Lancet* 356(9224):103–112.

UNAIDS (Joint United Nations Programme on HIV/AIDS). 2004. *2004 Report on the Global AIDS Epidemic: 4th Global Report.* Geneva, Switzerland: UNAIDS.

UNAIDS Global Reference Group on HIV/AIDS and Human Rights. 2004. *UNAIDS/WHO Policy Statement on HIV Testing.* Geneva, Switzerland: WHO.

Weinhardt LS, Carey MP, Johnson BT, Bickham NL. 1999. Effects of HIV counseling and testing on sexual risk behavior: A meta-analytic review of published research, 1985–1997. *American Journal of Public Health* 89(9):1397–1405.

WHO (World Health Organization). 2002. *World Health Organization ARV Toolkit.* [Online]. Available: http://www.who.int/hiv/toolkit/arv/en/content.jsp?ID=193&d=arv.06.01 [accessed March 10, 2005].

WHO. 2003a. *Emergency Scale-Up of Antiretroviral Therapy in Resource Limited Settings-Technical and Operational Recommendations to Achieve 3 by 5; Report of the WHO/UNAIDS International Congress Meeting on Technical and Operational Recommendations for Emergency Scaling-Up of Antiretroviral Therapy in Resource-Limited Settings.* Lusaka, Zambia, November 18–21, 2003.

WHO. 2003b. *Strategic Approaches to the Prevention of HIV Infections in Infants; Report of a WHO Meeting, Morges, Switzerland, March 20–22, 2002.* Geneva, Switzerland: WHO.

Wyss K. 2004a. *Scaling-Up Antiretroviral Treatment and Human Resources for Health: What Are the Challenges in Sub-Saharan Africa?* Berne, Switzerland: Swiss Agency for Development and Cooperation.

Wyss K. 2004b. *Human Resources for Health Development for Scaling-Up Antiretroviral Treatment in Tanzania.* Basel, Switzerland: Swiss Tropical Institute.

1

Introduction

Human beings are the heart of health care. It is their labor and their intellect that translate science and technology into healing and hope. Just as oils and brushes without painters cannot create art, drugs and diagnostics without health workers cannot create health care. Nowhere is this more evident today than in the fight against global HIV/AIDS, the greatest health crisis of our time. As of this writing in 2005, close to 40 million people harbor HIV, 95 percent of whom live in resource-poor areas. Even before the pandemic hit, the health systems in these areas were weak and under-staffed. Since the disease emerged, the dearth of health workers to treat and care for these HIV-infected individuals has reached crisis proportions.

The few health professionals practicing in many of the countries highly impacted by HIV/AIDS—workers often stressed, ill prepared, and scant in number—must now cope with a staggering new burden of disease while at the same time acquiring the knowledge, skills, and technology to deliver lifelong antiretroviral drug regimens, HIV/AIDS clinical and palliative care, and prevention services. Arguably, their task represents the most profound challenge in the scaling up of health care the world has ever known. They cannot accomplish this task alone.

This report explores potential strategies for mobilizing U.S. health personnel and technical experts to assist in the battle against HIV/AIDS in 15 African, Caribbean, and Southeast Asian countries highly affected by the disease. Commissioned by the U.S. Department of State as part of a historic global health initiative—the $15 billion 5-year President's Emergency Plan for AIDS Relief (PEPFAR), the report presents the results of a study conducted by the Institute of Medicine's Committee on the Options for Overseas Placement of U.S. Health Professionals.

STUDY CONTEXT

In his State of the Union address of January 28, 2003, President George W. Bush announced PEPFAR with three extraordinary goals: (1) providing antiretroviral therapy (ART) for 2 million people; (2) preventing 7 million new HIV infections; and (3) providing care to 10 million people infected with or affected by HIV/AIDS, including orphans and vulnerable children. On May 27, 2003, the U.S. Congress passed the United States Leadership against HIV/AIDS, Tuberculosis, and Malaria Act of 2003 (Public Law 108-25) to realize the President's vision. The act supports a phased expansion of critical programs, improved agency coordination, increased resources for multilateral and bilateral efforts, expansion of private-sector efforts, and intensified efforts to develop relevant HIV/AIDS therapies. Recognizing the contributions that U.S. health professionals can make in fighting HIV/AIDS, malaria, and tuberculosis in heavily affected, often resource-poor areas, the act also calls for a pilot program to demonstrate the feasibility of deploying U.S. personnel to such areas for periods of up to 3 years to provide basic health care services, deliver on-the-job training, and augment the health education of local populations. The legislation calls for a broad recruitment effort nationwide, including incentives such as loan repayment to encourage participation.

Without such reinforcement of human resources for health, PEPFAR's ambitious targets will be difficult if not impossible to achieve. Few African countries, for example, have more than one doctor per 5,000 persons; the number of physicians currently practicing is already insufficient to meet other needs without the additional burden of providing ART for the millions of medically eligible Africans now and over the next decade. The need for nurses and other health workers for ART scale-up is even more acute. In Uganda in 2005, for example, the projected ratio of diagnostic laboratory staff supporting ART scale-up to the annual output from in-country training institutions is roughly 10 to 1 (Adano et al., 2004). Pharmacists are similarly scarce. And assuming that all Ugandan nursing graduates worked on ART scale-up, there would still be a projected national shortfall of almost 2,000 nurses—roughly the same shortfall projected in South Africa, where major deficits of medical officers, pharmacists, dietitians, social workers, and counselors are also anticipated (South Africa Ministry of Health, 2003). In fact, comparable human resource needs—which do not even begin to address the larger agenda of HIV/AIDS counselling and testing, prevention of maternal-to-child transmission, and social and palliative care services—exist in virtually all of the 15 countries that are the focus of PEPFAR[1] (Adano et al., 2004).

Another factor exacerbating the human resource crisis in addressing global HIV/AIDS is the so-called "brain drain." Currently, many nurses and other health care workers trained in poor countries receive offers of employment in wealthier countries that are experiencing their own health care staffing shortages. A few examples begin to illustrate the dimensions of the problem. According to a report of the U.S. Agency for International Development (USAID) published in 2003, only 360 of the 1,200 doctors trained in Zimbabwe in the 1990s still practice domestically; in Zambia, only 50 of the 600 doctors trained locally since independence have remained in their country. Overall, many countries in sub-Saharan Africa have as many or fewer health workers today relative to 30 or even 40 years ago (JLI, 2004). The continued exodus of health personnel could seriously jeopardize ART scale-up.

Indigenous health professionals must be trained, supported, and retained if they are to be used to leverage and sustain the U.S. fiscal and human resource investment in services related to HIV/AIDS, including ART scale-up, as well as to other global health issues. The training of these professionals should encompass a wide range of clinical, social service, and administrative skills and values. Launching new, comprehensive health care delivery services that are effective and efficient will also require a mix of senior, midlevel, and junior professionals and suitably managed technical support. For example, laboratory assets must be well utilized and maintained and appropriately resourced with expendable supplies. Reliable drug delivery systems, along with education to maximize adherence, will be critical to prolong the durability of current treatment regimens. The treatment regimens themselves must be introduced at the optimal time in the natural history of the infection and appropriately monitored to reduce toxicity and the emergence of resistance. Experience has already shown that improper use of ART selects drug-resistant viruses. These strains, in turn, complicate the treatment of individuals while accelerating the spread of drug-resistant virus in the population as a whole, thus greatly increasing both the cost and complexity of HIV/AIDS care.

All of these lessons have already been learned over a 20-year history of comprehensive HIV/AIDS care in industrialized countries. A network of U.S. providers drawing on this experience should therefore have a positive

---

[1]Current PEPFAR focus countries are Botswana, Cote d'Ivoire, Ethiopia, Guyana, Haiti, Kenya, Mozambique, Namibia, Nigeria, Rwanda, South Africa, Tanzania, Uganda, Zambia, and Vietnam.

impact in fostering the most effective use of the U.S. dollars invested in PEPFAR and efforts in other developing countries.

Study Goals and Approach

This study was undertaken to provide a rapid, independent review of mechanisms for mobilizing the quantity and quality of relevant U.S. health personnel and technical experts needed in the 15 PEPFAR focus countries. In response to its charge, the committee explored both short- and long-term options for mobilizing, preparing, sending, managing, and compensating U.S. health professionals for service in these countries. Over its 7-month tenure, the committee:

- Reviewed available data sources to project the optimum size and composition of a U.S. global health professions service program to augment, train, and collaborate with the public health and clinical professionals already present in the host countries
- Assessed the relative strengths and weaknesses of existing and potential organizational models for such a program that could rapidly be activated or adapted to recruit, train, and place program participants
- Articulated principles that can be applied in evaluating the advantages and disadvantages of those models
- Examined other contextual issues bearing on the successful implementation of a U.S. global health professions service program

Committee members and consultants were selected for their international experience in low- and middle-income countries, as well as their individual expertise in the following areas relevant to the committee's charge: clinical medical practice; nursing; nongovernmental organizations and partnering; social science, health education, and training programs; pharmacy, logistics, and informatics; laboratory services in resource-constrained areas; administration and policy with regard to international health resources; epidemiology and operations research; academic health care; and faith-based organizations. A brief profile of each member and consultant can be found in Appendix H.

The committee convened twice between September 2004 and February 2005. The committee also cast a broad net to review relevant experience in mobilizing, preparing, sending, managing, and compensating U.S. health professionals willing to work overseas in developing countries. Testimony and data were presented at the committee's meetings and further discussed in frequent telephone conferences among subgroups, each consisting of three to six committee members and consultants. In addition, the committee reviewed and considered information from the published literature;

websites for governmental and nongovernmental organizations; and a variety of other sources, including four commissioned papers (see Appendixes B–E). The results of these efforts informed the committee in its preparation of this report.

BACKGROUND

Poverty and Health

Throughout history, poverty has plagued humankind. Today it remains the normal condition of life for at least a third of the world's population. Around 2.8 billion people worldwide live on less than $2 a day, while well over a billion subsist on less than $1 a day. As a consequence, almost everything that residents of wealthy countries take for granted—good nutrition, access to education, low rates of communicable disease, long life expectancies—is the exception rather than the rule for these global neighbors, whose daily reality often is characterized by unsafe drinking water, lack of sanitation, illiteracy, periodic food shortages, epidemic diseases, and premature death. One well-known economist alluded to the broad, ravaging effects of poverty when—advocating for greatly expanded health aid to the Third World—he observed that "millions of people . . . are dying from their poverty right now" (Africa Recovery, 2002:22).

The first preconditions for health that distinguish rich and poor nations are clean water and sanitation. In low-income countries today, more than 1.1 billion people lack safe drinking water, and another 2.4 billion lack access to sanitation (WHO and UNICEF, 2000). The resulting death toll, according to recent estimates of the World Health Organization (WHO), is 1.6 million people each year (WHO, 2004a).

A rich–poor gap can also be seen in childhood immunization. Almost 34 million infants each year still do not have access to basic immunization services, with the lowest coverage being found in sub-Saharan Africa. In 2001, of an estimated 745,000 deaths from measles (a disease that can be prevented with a single vaccine costing U.S. $0.26), more than half occurred in sub-Saharan Africa (WHO, 2002a).

In 2005, the three global scourges most interrelated with poverty are HIV/AIDS, malaria, and tuberculosis. Together they accounted for 5–7 million deaths (WHO, 2002b), and these diseases remain a major reason why the poor stay poor (Commission on Macroeconomics and Health, 2001). In other words, not only do HIV/AIDS, malaria, and tuberculosis target the poor, but in each case they also stunt economic growth and development in the communities and regions where they flourish.

How does one begin to battle the triple scourge of HIV/AIDS, malaria, and tuberculosis? Providing effective drugs to affected populations—albeit essential to any comprehensive strategy—is simply not enough. Each disease has unique and complex features that mandate knowledge and customized approaches to prevention, control, and clinical management. Thus without competent professionals to administer them and infrastructure to support their delivery, drugs alone do not equal life-saving health care.

By offering support and expertise to counterparts overseas and assisting in the training of new generations of desperately needed health workers, American health professionals can bring help and hope to those parts of the world where HIV/AIDS, malaria, and tuberculosis are laying the greatest waste to human life and spirit. In so doing, these "healers abroad" can also fight poverty and help sustain the long-term global health effort by multiplying essential skills and services. As citizens of a small world, we must acknowledge that in the end, such efforts benefit us all.

The Health Care Workforce and Global Health

Human Resources and Health[2]

Throughout history, human beings have driven health care (Anand and Barnighausen, 2004; World Bank, 1993). Health workers are active—not passive—agents of change. Often commanding two-thirds of today's health budgets, they link together the many parts of the health system to spearhead the provision of health care (Berman et al., 1999).

Why are health workers so important? A quick look at success stories in disease control—from yellow fever, hookworm, and smallpox eradication; to the child health revolution in the 1980s; to the imminent eradication of polio—reveals that all were built on human resource strategies. The formal, science-based education of physicians in the United States, first codified in the Flexner Report (Flexner, 1910), contributed to the doubling of life expectancy in the United States over the last century.

In a recent analysis of the global health care workforce, the Joint Learning Initiative—a consortium of more than 100 health leaders—argues that mobilizing and strengthening human resources will be central to combating health crises in some of the world's poorest countries and to building sustainable health systems in all countries (JLI, 2004). Yet nearly all nations today are challenged by worker shortages, skill mix imbalances, misdistribution of resources, negative work environments, and weak knowledge bases. This is particularly true in the poorest countries. In several of the most heavily impacted African countries, for example, the

---

[2]This section is drawn largely from the work of the Joint Learning Initiative (JLI, 2004).

prevalence of HIV among adults approaching 40 percent. The health sector is doubly affected by the HIV/AIDS epidemic: it must respond to the crippling burden of ill health among the general population while simultaneously dealing with the impact of the epidemic on health professionals. This situation represents the most profound change in the burden of disease ever experienced by any health system—much less those systems already weak and underfinanced before the advent of HIV/AIDS.

Added to this burden are new demands for diagnosis and treatment, including the challenges associated with provision of ART. Proper prescription of and monitoring of compliance with antiretroviral drug regimens are essential if patients are to benefit and if the grave possibility of emerging drug resistance is to be reduced. People living with HIV infection also require access to a wide range of care—from primary, secondary, and tertiary health care; to social services; to community-based support and home care.

Supervision and management skills and capacity are also critical to the effective delivery of all health care, including that focused on HIV/AIDS. In Tanzania and Chad, Kurowski and colleagues (2003) found evidence that improved staff management could result in substantial increases in staff productivity in the provision of HIV/AIDS care (Kurowski et al., 2003). Increased access to ART, voluntary counseling and testing, and prevention of mother-to-child transmission will require management as well as technical skills in relation to systems, administration, procurement, logistics, delivery, and referral; effective links between the formal and informal sectors will also be necessary. This challenge of good management is especially timely and pertinent within the broader contexts of decentralization and health-sector reform.

Despite general recognition of the crucial role of human resources in the provision of health care, the development of the health care workforce in low-income countries has suffered from years of national and international neglect (as discussed further below). Indeed, the dearth of qualified health care professionals in most low-income countries is the single most important constraint faced in responding to health care needs (Narasimhan et al., 2004). The Commission on Macroeconomics and Health, for example, has advocated a greatly increased investment in health, rising in low-income countries to a per capita expenditure of $34 per year. According to the commission, however, the main problem in implementing this recommendation is not the difficulty in raising the additional funds but the capacity of the health sector itself to absorb them (Habte et al., 2004). Likewise, senior officials in Ethiopia, Nigeria, and Uganda have all cited the lack of health care personnel as a main constraint in responding to health challenges (WHO AFRO, 2002). And Botswana, a comparatively rich African country that has committed to providing free ART to all eligible citizens, is hindered in doing so principally by a lack of health personnel (WHO, 2004b).

As new resources are being mobilized to fight HIV/AIDS, tuberculosis, malaria, and other global diseases, the health workforce crisis—especially in Africa—is daily becoming more apparent and dire. External grants and funding to address global HIV/AIDS, estimated at $5 billion in 2003, could reach $20 billion by 2007 (UNAIDS, 2004). At present, however, there is simply insufficient human capacity in many developing countries to absorb, apply, and make efficient use of these new funds and critical health initiatives.

The Current Global Health Care Workforce

> After a century of the most spectacular health advances in human history, we confront unprecedented and interlocking health crises. Some of the world's poorest countries face rising death rate and plummeting life expectancy, even as global pandemics threaten us all. Human survival gains are being lost because of feeble national health systems. On the front line of human survival, we see overburdened and overstressed health workers, too few in number, without the support they so badly need—losing the fight. Many are collapsing under strain; many are dying, especially from AIDS; and many are seeking a better life and more reward work by departing for richer countries (Chen et al., 2004).

According to statistics compiled by WHO, the world had 9 million doctors and 15 million nurses in 2000 (WHO, 2004c), representing an average density of 1.6 doctors and 2.5 nurses per 1,000 population. When compared with the results of the last published global survey in 1971 (which estimated a pool of 2.3 million doctors worldwide), the 2000 data suggest that the global supply of doctors is growing, on average, about 5 percent per year (Mejia and Pizurki, 1976). The total global health workforce is currently estimated at more than 100 million—a figure that includes 24 million recorded doctors, nurses, and midwives, plus another pool of uncounted informal, traditional, community, and allied workers (Chen et al., 2004).

These numbers do not tell the whole story, however. There is an extreme imbalance in the distribution of credentialed professionals among regions and countries. The supply of nurses and doctors relative to the population of sub-Saharan Africa, for instance, is one-tenth of that in Europe. To take an even more extreme case, Ethiopia has one-fiftieth of Italy's supply of health professionals (Chen et al., 2004).

Many factors contribute to this global imbalance in individual settings, but Chen and colleagues (2004) point to three major macro faced by assailing health workers: (1) the triple impact of HIV/AIDS, which, as noted above, increases the workloads of health care workers and exposes them to infection, while also stressing their morale (see Box 1-1) (Tawfik and Kinoti, 2003); (2) increased worker labor migration, depleting nurses and doctors from countries that can least afford the loss (as discussed in detail below) (Alkire and Chen, 2004); and (3) chronic underinvestment in human resources stemming from two decades of economic and sectoral reform that capped expenditures, froze recruitment and salaries, and restricted public budgets, thereby depleting working environments of basic supplies, drugs, and facilities (Narasimhan et al., 2004).

Educational systems of developing countries are another major impediment to the ongoing production of health workers. Europe produces 173,800 doctors a year, and Africa only 5,100 (JLI, 2004) (see Figure 1-1). One doctor is produced for every 5,000 people in Central and Eastern Europe and the Baltic States, compared with one doctor for every 115,000 people in sub-Saharan Africa. Moreover, in many health professions schools in developing countries, curricula are misaligned with prevailing patterns of disease, and teaching methods do not emphasize the practical problem-solving skills needed to address local health issues (Ndumbe, 2004). Instead of working competencies, production of health professionals is based on certification or Western medical standards. The result is a greater proportion of graduates focused on professional status and income generation, which further increases potential out-migration to wealthier countries.

The production of public health specialists is also insufficient in areas where these workers are most needed, leading to another critical disparity between rich and poor countries. A recent survey, for example, found that more than half of countries in Africa had no graduate training program in public health (Ijsselmuiden, 2003).

In many countries, including those with high HIV prevalence, the inability to recruit and retain an effective, well-motivated, appropriately skilled workforce stems from a range of additional problems that include low pay, poor work conditions, and weak management. Some workers experience a triple bind: their workplaces are understaffed and their compensation packages woefully inadequate, but civil service or public expenditure reforms prevent recruitment of new staff or substitutes for missing colleagues (sometimes called "ghost workers"). In recent years, these factors have fueled the trends for some health professionals to move from the public to the private sector or to leave their professions altogether, as well as the above-noted trend to migrate internationally in pursuit of more favorable opportunities.

The most common grievance of health workers is poor pay. Wages are often insufficient to cover personal and family needs. In addition, salaries may not be adjusted for rising inflation and may not be paid on time. In

BOX 1-1
The Triple Impact of HIV/AIDS on Health Workers

Increased Workload

Longitudinal hospital-based surveys in HIV-endemic areas confirm the rising inpatient burden of HIV/AIDS since the early days of the epidemic. Arthur and colleagues (2000, 2001) describe a steady rise in HIV-infected patients admitted to Kenyatta National Hospital, Nairobi, from 4.3 per day in 1988 to 13.9 in 1997. The rise in bed occupancy over the same period was 190 percent, plateauing at 40 percent HIV-positive census.

A recent report of the U.K. Department for International Development (DFID, 2003) estimates the current bed occupancy at Kenyatta National Hospital even higher, at 300 percent, 70 percent HIV-related. The report also states that 50 percent of bed occupancy in Eldoret, Kenya, is HIV-related, and 75 percent of Eldoret's tuberculosis (TB) patients are coinfected with HIV. In KwaZulu Natal, South Africa, hospital admissions rose by 81 percent over 10 years, while adult TB admissions (an indirect reflection of the HIV/AIDS burden) rose by 360 percent, accounting for 47 percent of male and 30 percent of female medical ward admissions and 11 percent of total hospital admissions (Floyd et al., 1999).

According to the 2001 Swaziland Human Development Report, people with HIV occupied 50 percent of the beds in some health care centers (DFID, 2003). In Zimbabwe, HIV prevalence among hospitalized patients also rose to 50 percent, making HIV the leading cause of hospitalization. A study in Tanzania found that patients with HIV had three times the average length of stay of non-HIV patients (18 versus 6 days); two Tanzanian district hospitals had to construct new wards to cope with the increasing demand for HIV-related care (Malecela-Lazaro et al., 2001).

Against this backdrop of growing HIV/AIDS-related inpatient burdens, Tawfik and Kinoti (2003) note that only scanty, mainly anecdotal information exists regarding the impact of the epidemic on individual health professionals (Tawfik and Kinoti, 2003). It is clear, however, that HIV/AIDS brings increasing and changing workloads, often demanding higher skills (especially with the introduction of ART). Recent modeling of human resources for health in Tanzania and Chad suggests that many tasks and activities are carried out by staff not formally qualified to perform them, and that surpluses of staff with lower skills must compensate for deficits of staff with higher skills (Kurowski et al., 2003). China, a country where more than 1 million people in rural areas have contracted HIV through unsafe blood collection procedures, is experiencing difficulties in providing ART because of the shortage of doctors with the necessary training and skills (Sui, 2003).

Along with increased workload, health workers in areas highly impacted by HIV/AIDS must cope with new roles for which they are neither trained nor equipped—in particular, the psychosocial support of patients and families facing the emotional trauma of the disease. Finally, HIV has a negative effect on staff productivity through absenteeism related to caring for ill relatives and attending funerals.

Exposure to HIV Infection

While individual health workers are generally subject to the same risks of acquiring HIV/AIDS as the general population, they may also risk infection in the course of caring for HIV-infected and other patients. This occupational risk of infection varies between developed and resource-poor countries and across health worker categories. A study in a South African hospital investigating the potential for HIV transmission from needle sticks and other sharp-instrument injuries found that 41 percent of such injuries occurred among nurses and 38 percent among cleaners, although the latter comprised only 16 percent of total hospital personnel (de Villiers, 2000). Nurses are probably at high risk overall. In just a few years, the HIV prevalence rate among nurses in Lusaka, Zambia, rose from 34 to 44 percent (Ndongko and Oladepo, 2003).

Health workers are also at risk of acquiring other infections in their workplaces, such as tuberculosis transmitted through respiratory secretions and additional blood-borne pathogens, such as hepatitis B and C, acquired through exposure to the blood and body fluids of carriers. In one study, the incidence of tuberculosis was found to have increased several-fold among health workers in areas with high HIV prevalence (Whiteside, 2002).

Husain and Badcock-Walters (2002) have estimated that a country with a stable 15 percent prevalence rate can expect between 1.6 percent and 3.3 percent of its health care providers to die from HIV/AIDS each year. As of 1999, it was estimated that in Botswana, 17 to 32 percent of health workers were HIV-infected, and between 28 and 41 percent would be infected by 2005. Malawi and Zambia have experienced five- to sixfold increase in illness and death rates among health workers. A recent report of the Joint United Nations Programme on HIV/AIDS (UNAIDS) suggests that training of doctors and nurses in southern Africa needs to increase by 25 to 40 percent by 2010 simply to compensate for these expected losses (UNAIDS, 2002).

Psychosocial Effects

HIV/AIDS has profound psychosocial impacts on health workers. In some cases, the epidemic raises workers' awareness of previously excluded social groups, while other health professionals either withdraw from or reject patients who are sex workers or intravenous drug users. Emotional reactions may also include exaggerated fears of exposure to HIV, homophobia, and other negative attitudes towards specific social groups, as well as cultural, social, or moral resistance to promoting certain HIV/AIDS preventive practices, such as the use of condoms. Tawfik and Kinoti (2003) and Malecela-Lazaro and colleagues (2001) underscore that feelings of professional inadequacy and hopelessness may partly explain poor work performance in some areas of high HIV/AIDS burden. For example, workers may believe that providing health care to dying HIV/AIDS victims is a waste of time and resources that could be used to treat and cure other patients.

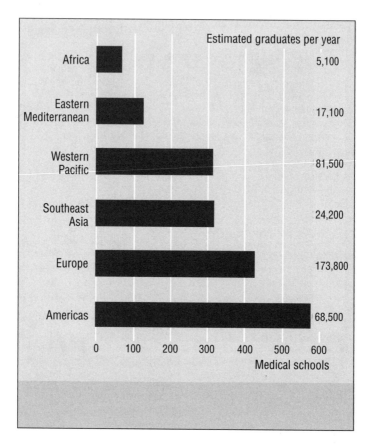

Estimated graduates per year

Region		Estimated graduates per year
Africa		5,100
Eastern Mediterranean		17,100
Western Pacific		81,500
Southeast Asia		24,200
Europe		173,800
Americas		68,500

Medical schools

FIGURE 1-1 Regional disparities in medical schools and graduates.
NOTE: Region refers to WHO regions.
SOURCE: Adapted from JLI (2004) and Eckhert (2002).

many countries, civil service wages have actually fallen in recent years. In Tanzania, a civil servant's wage in 1998 was only 70 percent of that in 1969 (JLI, 2004). Wages of registered nursed in Malawi when adjusted for the cost of living amount to about $489 a month (Vujicic et al., 2004). In Ghana and Zambia, the average monthly salary for a doctor is just over $400 (HLF, 2004).

Low wages in the public sector can also drive workers into "dual practices," whereby public servants provide private services (Ferrinho et al., 2004; Vujicic et al., 2004). Such practices are breeding grounds for professional and financial conflicts of interest as workers juggle their public obligations while attempting to maximize income from more lucrative assignments and services (often based in urban centers). In the worst case, inadequate compensation of health workers can lead to overtly predatory behavior—for example, marketing and selling of drugs, or demands for illegal payments for services.

Poor work environments also negatively impact retention and performance by workers in the health sector. Heavy workloads, burnout, excessive administrative duties, isolation from colleagues, lack of teamwork, and occupational hazards are additional reasons for low worker morale. Finally, a lack of recognition, a lack of career opportunities, and atmospheres that generally discourage creativity all serve to demotivate health workers who are already underpaid.

On the other hand, nonfinancial incentives—career advancement and continuing education, flexible work hours, good employment conditions, adequate vacation time, and access to child care—can increase worker motivation. Upgrading competencies, facilitating access to specialized training in the future, and accelerating promotion and career development can also be helpful in at least temporarily redressing geographic imbalances in the health care workforce. Indonesia and Thailand, for example, set aside specialist training slots for workers who have completed rural service in order to improve rural access to workers (Chomitz et al., 1998; Wibulpolprasert, 1999; Wibulpolprasert and Pengpaibon, 2003). South Africa and Malawi have used bonding or compulsory service regulations to shift their geographic distribution of health workers, although these methods have proven difficult to monitor and enforce (Chomitz et al., 1998; Hammer and Jack, 2002).

Goals for Achieving Global Health

At the Millennium Summit of the United Nations General Assembly in September 2000, delegates adopted an ambitious set of goals aimed at reducing global poverty, ignorance, and ill health over the next 15 years. Some goals had been proposed at earlier summits devoted to specific social problems, such as health and education, but never before had the United Nations backed such a comprehensive antipoverty agenda. The following seven goals were adopted:

- Halving the proportion of people who live in extreme poverty and the proportion of people in hunger over the period 1990–2015
- Achieving universal primary education for both boys and girls by 2015
- Promoting gender equality and the empowerment of women
- Reducing child (under age 5) mortality by two-thirds between 1990 and 2015

• Reducing maternal mortality by three-quarters between 1990 and 2015

• Halting and beginning to reverse the spread of HIV/AIDS, malaria, and other major diseases by 2015

• Integrating principles of environmental sustainability into national development goals

The density of health workers in a given country will make an enormous difference to the likelihood that its population will meet specific indicators for the health-related goals listed above. For example, the prospects for achieving 80 percent coverage of measles immunization and skilled attendants at birth are much higher in countries where worker density exceeds 2.5 per 1,000 population. Seventy-five countries with 2.5 billion people currently fall below this minimum threshold (JLI, 2004).

Anand and Barnighausen (2004) conducted a quantitative cross-national analysis of human resource density and health status in 118 countries for which data were available. Not surprisingly, lower maternal, infant, and under-5 mortality rates were associated with higher income, higher female adult literacy, and lower poverty. After controlling for these expected findings, however, the analysis also showed that human resource density (physicians, nurses, and midwives per 1,000 population) mattered significantly in determining health outcome measures. Specifically, the authors found that as the density of health workers increased, maternal, infant, and under-5 mortality fell (see Figure 1-2). Maternal mortality was most sensitive to health worker density: a 10 percent increase in the density of the health workforce was correlated with a 4 percent decline in maternal mortality. A 10 percent increase in health worker density was correlated with a 2 percent decline in under-5 mortality.[3]

Achieving the above goals for health will therefore require concerted efforts to increase the total health workforce in developing countries. The Joint Learning Initiative estimates that sub-Saharan African countries must nearly triple their current health workforce by adding the equivalent of 1 million workers through retention, recruitment, and training if they are to come close to meeting these goals (Chen et al., 2004).

---

[3]Why is there a stronger effect on maternal mortality? A reasonable hypothesis is that highly trained medical personnel are more essential for the emergency obstetrical services needed to avert maternal deaths than for simpler tasks, such as immunization and treatment of common respiratory and intestinal infections, associated with infant and child health care.

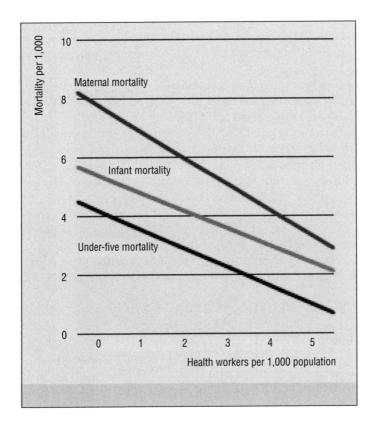

FIGURE 1-2 More health workers, fewer deaths.
SOURCE: Adapted from JLI (2004) and Anand and Barnighausen (2004).
Reprinted, with permission, from Elsevier (*The Lancet* 2004:1606).

The Health Workforce Crisis in Africa[4]

The problem of insufficient human resources for health care is most acute in sub-Saharan Africa, which bears 25 percent of the world's burden of disease but houses only 1.3 percent of the world's health workforce. Currently, an estimated 750,000 health workers serve the 682 million people of sub-Saharan Africa. The ratio of health care workers to population is 10 to 15 times higher in countries of the Organization for Economic Cooperation and Development (OECD) (HLF, 2004).

---

[4]This section is drawn largely from the work of the High-Level Forum on the Health Millennium Development Goals (2004).

The High-Level Forum on the Health Millennium Development Goals (2004) identifies four major factors contributing to the low density of health workers in Africa compared with other regions of the world:

- Insufficient training opportunities—Two-thirds of sub-Saharan African countries have only one medical school, and 11 sub-Saharan African countries have no medical school (Hagopian et al., 2004).
- Deteriorating health of the workforce—The International Labor Organization has suggested that 18 to 41 percent of the workforce in many countries of sub-Saharan Africa is infected with HIV-1 (Cohen, 2002).
- Rural/urban imbalance—In Tanzania, the city of Dar-es-Salaam alone has nearly 30 times as many medical officers and medical specialists as other rural districts (Wyss, 2004). Only about 5 of Uganda's roughly 100 surgeons work outside of urban areas (Wasike, 2003). A 2003 USAID report notes that only one-fourth of rural doctors in South Africa are South African nationals, with most of the remainder coming from other African countries, such as Zambia, Zimbabwe, and Congo (Kober and Van Damme, 2004).
- The transnational flow of health professionals, or the "brain drain"— The international migration of health workers is discussed in greater detail in the following section. However, the High Level Forum anticipates that still-rising investments in health by OECD countries (projected to increase 10-fold over the next 50 years) (Chen, 2004) will continue to fuel the exodus of African health workers to wealthy countries if countermeasures are not taken.

A quick comparison of selected categories of health care providers in the 15 countries currently targeted by PEPFAR reveals a wide range of available providers in 2004 (see Table 1-1). By comparison, the current U.S. ranges as of October 2004 are shown in Table 1-2. The estimated gap in the total number of nurses, doctors, and midwives for the 15 PEPFAR focus countries, based on a minimum density of 2.5 doctors, nurses, and midwives per 1,000 population, is presented in Table 1-3.

International Migration of Health Care Workers

Of the 175 million people (2.9 percent of the world's population) living outside the country of birth in 2000, 65 million were economically active. The rise in the number of people migrating is significant for many developing countries because they are losing their better-educated nationals to richer countries. Medical practitioners and nurses represent a small proportion of the highly skilled workers who migrate, but the loss for devel-

TABLE 1-1 Health Care Providers (per 100,000 Population) in Selected PEPFAR Countries

Providers	Low	High
Physicians	1.9 (Rwanda)	69.0 (South Africa)
Nurses and Midwives	8.8 (Uganda)	388.0 (South Africa)
Dentists	0.05 (Rwanda)	10.5 (South Africa)
Pharmacists	0.1 (Rwanda)	24.2 (South Africa)

SOURCE: WHO (2004c).

TABLE 1-2 Health Care Providers (per 100,000 Population) in the United States

Providers	Number
Physicians	293
Nurses and Midwives	773
Dentists	59
Pharmacists	69

SOURCE: WHO (2004c).

oping countries of human resources in the health sector may mean that the capacity of the health system to deliver health care equitably is significantly compromised. It is unlikely that migration will stop given the advances in global communications and the development of global labor markets in some fields, which now include nursing (Stilwell et al., 2004).

The migration of health personnel across international borders is having major negative impacts on health systems in developing countries. Migration is currently possible for all health professionals who have marketable skills. Despite temporary declines in demand from recipient countries, overall demand for health professionals has increased since the 1970s, facilitated by globalized markets and free-trade agreements that have reduced barriers to trade and to the mobility of services, products, and people (Martineau et al., 2004). Although the migration of doctors receives the most attention, it is the movement of nurses and other health professionals that can cripple a health system. Nurses are in particularly high demand for aging populations in wealthy countries, and are proactively recruited by professional firms through enticements of 10-fold or greater salary differentials (Narasimhan et al., 2004). This migration, a consequence of globaliza-

TABLE 1-3 Deficit or Surplus of Doctors, Nurses, and Midwives

PEPFAR Countries	Population (in thousands)	Doctors, Nurses, and Midwives per 1,000 Population	Surplus/Deficit[a]
Guyana	759	2.77	+200
Haiti	7,797	0.36	−16,700
Vietnam	79,197	1.28	−96,600
Ethiopia	68,961	0.23	−156,500
Botswana	1,697	2.70	+300
Cote d'Ivoire	14,685	0.55	−28,600
Kenya	27,390	1.03	−40,300
Mozambique	17,861	0.31	−39,100
Namibia	1,750	3.14	+1100
Nigeria	114,746	1.45	−120,500
Rwanda	8,273	0.23	−18,800
South Africa	44,416	4.57	+91,900
Tanzania	36,276	0.39	−76,500
Uganda	25,004	0.14	−59,000
Zambia	9,371	1.20	−12,200
TOTAL			−571,300

[a]Actual number rounded to nearest hundred.
NOTE: Human Resources in Health (HRH) density of 2.5 doctors, nurses, and midwives per 1,000 population.
SOURCE: JLI (2004).

tion, is one of the priority issues being addressed by mode 4 of the General Agreement on Trade in Services.

The following examples illustrate the problem:

• There are reportedly more Malawian doctors in Manchester, England, than in Malawi (JLI, 2004).

• Only 50 of 600 Zambian doctors trained since independence continue to practice in that country (WHO, 2004d).

• Doctors in the Philippines are retraining themselves as nurses to pursue lucrative overseas opportunities (Chan, 2003).

• In 2001, 382 nurses migrated from Zimbabwe to the United Kingdom, increasing the latter country's nursing stock by only 0.1 percent but depleting Zimbabwe's available pool by 4 percent (Buchan and Dovlo, 2004).

• In South Africa, the national HIV/AIDS treatment plan aims to create 12,000 new posts, yet 29,000 positions in the public health sector are currently unfilled. More than 82,000 health workers left South Africa between 1989 and 1997 (Cohen, 2002).

Migration can also affect key services or regions. Wholesale recruitment of the nursing staff of an intensive care unit (ICU) at a hospital in the Philippines essentially cut off access to ICU care for the local population (BBC News, 2003). And the migration of service workers from Malawi to the United Kingdom is leading to the near collapse of maternity service in Malawi's central hospital (Dugger, 2004).

Currently, foreign doctors can make up as much as a third of the total number of doctors in developed countries (see Figure 1-3). Migration patterns are generated by "push" and "pull" factors facilitated by labor markets, language compatibility, sociocultural affinities, professional equivalency, and visa policies. Six principal factors driving these movements are job satisfaction, career opportunity, governance and management, safety and risks, and social and family reasons (Dovlo and Martineau, 2004).

One way to address this problem is to promote "reverse flows" (JLI, 2004). Box 1-2 describes one such attempt. Innovative strategies include volunteer cadres, expansion of nongovernmental activities, and north–south institutional twinning or partnerships. Exporting countries—for example, Cuba, Egypt, India, and the Philippines—could also accelerate their flows to countries with severe health workforce shortages. Cuba already provides significant human resources to many African and Caribbean nations, while at present, the other three countries target primarily richer, OECD countries (JLI, 2004).

From the broadest perspective, what is needed today is global responsibility and collaboration to slow the pace of doctors and nurses following multiple entry and exit paths from low- to high-income countries. As the Joint Learning Initiative report states, "no country is an island in workforce development." The report further indicates that migratory flows produce benefits as well as harm, and blocking the movement of people violates human rights and is generally unenforceable. "[Therefore], the global management of medical migration should seek to protect both health and human rights—dampening 'push' forces by retaining talent in sending countries and reducing 'pull' forces by aiming for educational and workforce self-sufficiency in destination countries" (JLI, 2004:6).

ORGANIZATION OF THE REPORT

In this report, the committee proposes a set of interconnected workforce enhancement programs that would meet the need to augment the health professionals currently waging the fight against HIV/AIDS and other global diseases. The committee believes that, given adequate resources, talent, and political will, these programs would make an enormous contribution to the eventual control of these terrible afflictions.

The report is organized into two parts (see Box 1-3). The first part

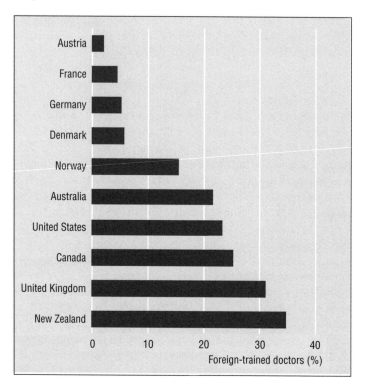

FIGURE 1-3 Percentage of foreign-trained doctors in selected developed countries. NOTE: Data are for 1998 for Australia and Canada; 2000 for France, Germany, and New Zealand; 2001 for Austria, the United Kingdom, and the United States; 2002 for Norway. Figures shown for Austria represent physicians that have obtained recognition of their qualifications in Austria; for France, as a percentage of the medical workforce in France; Germany as a percentage of the active medical workforce in Germany; for Australia as a percentage of the employed medical workforce in Australia; for New Zealand, as a percentage of the active medical practitioners in New Zealand.
SOURCE: Adapted from JLI (2004) and OECD (2002).
Data adapted from www.oecd.org/dac/stats/crs, © OECD, All rights reserved.

reviews and provides evidence for the current human resource crisis in global health, outlines the challenges of confronting HIV/AIDS (and other global diseases) on the ground, and describes a range of national and international initiatives currently focused on global HIV/AIDS. The second part begins by presenting the philosophy and guiding principles of the master government program—the Global Health Service—envisioned by the com-

BOX 1-2
Reversing the Brain Drain: TOKTEN in Vietnam

The Transfer of Knowledge through Expatriate Nationals (TOKTEN) program was launched by the United Nations Development Program (UNDP) in 1977 as an attempt to reverse patterns of brain drain by encouraging expatriate nationals to volunteer their expertise in the service of their homelands for short periods of time. The program is currently instituted in more than 25 countries, including Vietnam. Through this program, highly skilled expatriate professionals provide technical expertise, policy advice, and research to governments, private- and public-sector enterprises, universities, and research centers in various fields. TOKTEN consultants are considered volunteers, although UNDP covers travel expenses to and from the participant's country of residence and provides a generous stipend for living costs.

Under the program, qualified expatriate professionals from developing nations return to their countries of origin for typically 1 to 6 months to share the skills they have gained during their residence in developed countries. TOKTEN consultants carry out tasks that might otherwise be performed by international consultants, their volunteering often being motivated by the desire to play a role in the development of their country of origin. Transfer of knowledge occurs at a much lower cost than is the case with foreign consultants (often with savings of 50–70 percent) and more rapidly as well, since TOKTEN consultants need no period of adjustment to become acquainted with the language or the social and cultural context. In virtually all cases, networks are created, and follow-up takes place.

TOKTEN was first initiated in Vietnam in 1989, and in the decade since, two projects that include TOKTEN recruitment have been completed. The first TOKTEN project developed a roster of 194 potential expatriate consultants and established relationships between Vietnamese organizations and the organization of each fielded consultant. Between 1990 and 1992, 60 requests for consultants were received, and 20 TOKTEN consultants were placed. The first TOKTEN project was focused mainly in the area of science and technology. The receiving organizations included the Institute for Scientific and Technological Strategic Studies, Institute for Medical Equipment, Ben Tre Committee for Sciences, Institute for Computer Science, and Hanoi Polytechnic. TOKTEN volunteers in Vietnam receive a monthly living allowance with additional amounts given for up to two dependents.

SOURCE: Adapted from http://www.papp.undp.org/governance/projects/ and http://www.undp.org.vn/mlist/develvn/042001/post76.htm.

mittee as the primary vehicle for a new suite of programs designed to address the global HIV/AIDS workforce crisis and help achieve the PEPFAR goals. It then provides detailed descriptions of six proposed programs of the Global Health Service, along with short- and long-term mechanisms for mobilizing, preparing, sending, managing, and compensating U.S. health professionals serving in the PEPFAR focus countries. The last chapter of the

BOX 1-3
Report Organization

The Human Resource Crisis in Global Health

Chapter 1   Introduction
Chapter 2   Confronting HIV/AIDS on the Ground
Chapter 3   New Routes of Engagement against Global HIV/AIDS

Americans Responding to the Crisis

Chapter 4   Envisioning a U.S. Global Health Service
Chapter 5   Programs of the U.S. Global Health Service
Chapter 6   Looking Ahead

report revisits the big picture of national health capacity development in resource-poor and other countries; value-added investments in achieving the PEPFAR goals; ethical issues in foreign workforce assistance; creative public–private partnerships and alliances under PEPFAR; and processes for monitoring, evaluation, and adjustment.

REFERENCES

Adano U, O'Neil M, Decima E, Kiarie W. 2004. *Rapid Assessment of the Human Resource Implications of Scaling Up HIV/AIDS Services in Uganda.* Management and Leadership Development Project/USAID. Boston, MA: Management Sciences for Health.

Africa Recovery, United Nations. 2002. To cure poverty, heal the poor. *Africa Recovery* 16(1):22.

Alkire S, Chen L. 2004. *"Medical Exceptionalism" in International Migration: Should Doctors and Nurses Be Treated Differently?* Joint Learning Initiative Working Paper 7-3. [Online]. Available: http://www.globalhealthtrust.org/doc/abstracts/WG7/Alkirepaper.pdf [accessed February 8, 2005].

Anand S, Barnighausen T. 2004. Human resources and health outcomes: Cross-country econometric study. *Lancet* 364(9445):1603–1609.

Arthur G, Bhatt SM, Muhindi D, Achiya GA, Kariuki SM, Gilks CF. 2000. The changing impact of HIV/AIDS on Kenyatta National Hospital, Nairobi from 1988/89 through 1992 to 1997. *AIDS* 14(11):1625–1631.

Arthur G, Nduba VN, Kariuki SM, Kimari J, Bhatt SM, Gilks CF. 2001. Trends in bloodstream infections among human immunodeficiency virus-infected adults admitted to a hospital in Nairobi, Kenya, during the last decade. *Clinical Infectious Diseases* 33(2):248–256.

BBC News. 2003, August 27. *Nurses Exodus.* [Online]. Available: http://news.bbc.co.uk/2/hi/programmes/newsnight/3184479.stm [accessed March 4, 2005].

Berman P, Arellanes L, Henderson P, Magnoli A. 1999. *Health Care Financing in Eight Latin American and Caribbean Nations: The First Regional National Health Accounts Network.* Partners for Health Reform-LAC-HSR Paper N. 16.

Buchan J, Dovlo D. 2004. *International Recruitment of Health Workers to the UK: A Report to DFID*. London, England: DFID Health Systems Resource Centre.

Chan D. 2003. *Philippine Doctors Study Nursing to Land US Jobs*. [Online]. Available: http://www.sikhspectrum.com/032003/p_doctors.htm [accessed March 23, 2005].

Chen L. 2004. *Harnessing the Power of Human Resources for Achieving the MDGs*. Presentation at the January 9, 2004, Meeting of the High Level Forum on the Health Millennium Development Goals. Geneva, Switzerland.

Chen L, Evans T, Anand S, Boufford JI, Brown H, Chowdhury M, Cueto M, Dare L, Dussault G, Elzinga G, Fee E, Habte D, Hanvoravongchai P, Jacobs M, Kurowski C, Michael S, Pablos-Mendez A, Sewankambo N, Solimano G, Stilwell B, de Waal A, Wibulpolprasert S. 2004. Human resources for health: Overcoming the crisis. *Lancet* 364(9449):1984–1990.

Chomitz KM, Setiardi G, Azwar A, Ismail N. 1998. *What Do Doctors Want? Developing Incentives for Doctors to Serve in Indonesia's Rural and Remote Areas, Working Paper*. Washington, DC: World Bank.

Cohen D. 2002. *Human Capital and the HIV Epidemic in sub-Saharan Africa, Working Paper 2*. Geneva, Switzerland: International Labour Organization.

Commission on Macroeconomics and Health. 2001. *Macroeconomics and Health: Investing in Health for Economic Development*. Geneva, Switzerland: WHO.

de Villiers A. 2000 (July 7–12). *Abstract TuPeD3637: Retrospective Analysis of Injury on Duty Cases with Specific Emphasis on HIV Transmission as Reported in a Secondary Hospital in Bleomfontein, South Africa*. Presented at the XIII International AIDS Conference, Durban, South Africa.

DFID (U.K. Department for International Development) Health Systems Resource Centre. 2003. *Scoping Study on the Impact of HIV/AIDS on Health Systems*. London, England: DFID and John Snow International. [Online]. Available: http://www.jsiuk.com/docs/hiv_impact_study.pdf [accessed March 1, 2005].

Dovlo D, Martineau T. 2004. *Review of Evidence for Push and Pull Factors and Impact on Health Worker Mobility in Africa*. Joint Learning Initiative Working Paper. Ghana and Liverpool School of Tropical Medicine, United Kingdom.

Dugger C. 2004, July 12. An exodus of African nurses puts infants and the ill in peril. *The New York Times*. P. A1.

Eckhert N. 2002. The global pipeline: Too narrow, too wide, or just right? *Medical Education* 36(7):606–613.

Ferrinho P, Lerberghe WV, Fronteira I, Hipolito F, Biscaia A. 2004. *Dual Practice in the Health Sector: A Review of Evidence*. Joint Learning Initiative Working Paper. [Online]. Available: http://globalhealthtrust.org/doc/abstracts/WG3/Ferrinhoabstract.pdf [accessed March 1, 2005].

Flexner A. 1910. *Medical Education in the United States and Canada: A Report to the Carnegie Foundation for the Advancement of Teaching*. New York, NY: Carnegie Foundation for the Advancement of Teaching.

Floyd K, Reid RA, Wilkinson D, Gilks CF. 1999. Admission trends in a rural South African hospital during the early years of the HIV epidemic. *Journal of the American Medical Association* 282(11):1087–1091.

Habte D, Dussault G, Dovlo D. 2004. Challenges confronting the health workforce in sub-Saharan Africa. *World Hospitals & Health Services* 40(2):23–26, 40–41.

Hagopian A, Thompson M, Fordycel M, Johnson K, Hart LG. 2004. The migration of physicians from sub-Saharan Africa to the United States of America: Measures of the African brain drain. *Human Resources for Health* 2(17).

Hammer J, Jack W. 2002. Designing incentives for rural health care providers in developing countries. *Journal of Development Economics* 69(1):297–303.

HLF (High Level Forum on the Health Millennium Development Goals). 2004. *Addressing Africa's Health Workforce Crisis: An Avenue for Action.* Abuja, Nigeria: World Bank and WHO.

Husain I, Badcock-Walters P. 2002. HIV/AIDS, health and education. In: Forsythe S, ed. *State of the Art: AIDS and Economics.* Washington, DC: Policy Project and Merck and Co. Inc. Pp. 84–95.

Ijsselmuiden C. 2003 (September 29–October 3). *Training of Health Care Workers. Graduate Education in Public Health: Afri-Health Survey: Provisional Results and Conclusions.* Prepared for the Joint Learning Initiative, Accra Ghana.

JLI (Joint Learning Initiative). 2004. *Human Resources for Health: Overcoming the Crisis.* Cambridge, MA: Harvard University Press.

Kober K, Van Damme W. 2004. Scaling up access to antiretroviral treatment in southern Africa: Who will do the job? *Lancet* 364(9428):103–107.

Kurowski C, Wyss K, Abdulla S, Yemadji N, Mills A. 2003. *Human Resources for Health: Requirements and Availability in the Context of Scaling-Up Priority Interventions in Low-Income Countries: Case Studies from Tanzania and Chad.* London, England: London School of Hygiene and Tropical Medicine.

Malecela-Lazaro M, Mwisongo A, Makundi E, Mubyazi G, Kisinza W, Senkoro K, Magesa S, Malebo H, Mcharo J, Hiza P, Pallangyo, Ipuge Y, Kitua A. 2001. *HIV/AIDS Impact on Health Services in Tanzania.* Dar-es-Salaam, Tanzania: National Institute for Medical Research Health Systems and Policy Research Department.

Martineau T, Decker K, Bundred P. 2004. "Brain drain" of health professionals: From rhetoric to responsible action. *Health Policy* 70(1):1–10.

Mejia A, Pizurki H. 1976. World migration of health manpower. *WHO Chronicle* 30(11): 455–460.

Narasimhan V, Brown H, Pablos-Mendez A, Adams O, Dussault G, Elzinga G, Nordstrom A, Habte D, Jacobs M, Solimano G, Sewankambo N, Wibulpolprasert S, Evans T, Chen L. 2004. Responding to the global human resources crisis. *Lancet* 363(9419):1469–1472.

Ndongko W, Oladepo O. 2003. *Impact of HIB/AIDS on Public Sector Capacity in sub-Saharan Africa: Towards a Framework for the Protection of Public Sector Capacity and Effective Response to the Most Affected Countries.* Africa Capacity Building Foundation, Board of Governors. 13th Annual Meeting, June 29, 2004, The Hague.

Ndumbe P. 2004. *The Training of Human Resources for Health in Africa.* Joint Learning Initiative Working Paper 4-1. [Online]. Available: http://www.globalhealthtrust.org/doc/abstracts/WG4/NdumbeHRHFINAL.pdf [accessed March 1, 2005].

OECD (Organization for Economic Cooperation and Development). 2002. *International Migration of Physicians and Nurses: Causes, Consequences, and Health Policy Implications.* Draft. Paris, France: OECD.

South Africa Ministry of Health. 2003. *Operational Plan for Comprehensive HIV and AIDS Care, Management and Treatment for South Africa.* Pretoria, South Africa: South Africa Department of Health.

Stilwell B, Diallo K, Zurn P, Vujicic M, Adams O, Dal Poz M. 2004. Migration of health-care workers from developing countries: Strategic approaches to its management. *Bulletin of the World Health Organization* 8:596–600.

Sui C. 2003, July 15. *China–AIDS: China Starts Offering Free AIDS Drugs but Lacks Doctors to Administer Them.* Paris, France: Agence France-Presse. [Online]. Available: http://www.aegis.com/news/afp/2003/AF030781.html [accessed March 4, 2005].

Tawfik L, Kinoti S. 2003. *The Impact of HIV/AIDS on the Health Workforce in sub-Saharan Africa: The Issue of Human Resources: Support for Analysis and Research in Africa Project (SARA).* Washington, DC: USAID.

UNAIDS (Joint United Nations Programme on HIV/AIDS). 2002. *2002 Report on the Global AIDS Epidemic*. Geneva, Switzerland: UNAIDS.

UNAIDS. 2004. *2004 Report on the Global AIDS Epidemic: 4th Global Report*. Geneva, Switzerland: UNAIDS.

USAID (United States Agency for International Development). 2003. *The Health Sector Human Resource Crisis in Africa: An Issues Paper*. Washington, DC: USAID.

Vujicic M, Zurn P, Diallo K, Adams O, Dal Poz MR. 2004. The role of wages in the migration of health care professionals from developing countries. *Human Resources for Health* 2(1):3.

Wasike A. 2003, December 4. Go to the rural areas, PM tells medics. *New Vision, Uganda*.

Whiteside A. 2002. HIV/AIDS, health and education. In: Forsythe S, ed. *State of the Art: AIDS and Economics*. Washington, DC: Policy Project and Merck and Co. Inc. Pp. 24–29.

WHO (World Health Organization). 2002a. *World Health Report 2002: Reducing Risks, Promoting Healthy Life*. Geneva, Switzerland: WHO.

WHO. 2002b. *Report on Infectious Diseases: Scaling-Up the Response to Infectious Diseases*. Geneva, Switzerland: WHO.

WHO. 2004a. *Investment in Water and Sanitation Yields Health and Economic Benefits*. [Online]. Available: http://www.who.int/mediacentre/news/releases/2004/pr28/en/ [accessed March 1, 2005].

WHO. 2004b. *Summary Country Profile for HIV/AIDS Treatment Scale-Up: Botswana*. [Online]. Available: http://www.who.int/3by5/en/cp_bwa.pdf [accessed March 1, 2005].

WHO. 2004c. *Global Atlas of the Health Workforce*. [Online]. Available: http://www.who.int/GlobalAtlas/DataQuery/home.asp [accessed March 1, 2005].

WHO. 2004d. *Human Resources for Health Country Synthesis*. Geneva, Switzerland: WHO.

WHO AFRO (Regional Office for Africa). 2002. *Report on Consultative Meeting on Improving Collaboration Between Health Professionals, Governments, and Other Stakeholders in Human Resources for Health Development*. Addis Ababa, Ethiopia: WHO. [Online]. Available: http://www.afro.who.int/hrd/consultative_meeting_report.pdf [accessed March 1, 2005].

WHO and UNICEF (World Health Organization and United Nations Children's Fund). 2000. *Global Water Supply and Sanitation Assessment 2000 Report*. Geneva, Switzerland: Joint Monitoring Programme for Water Supply and Sanitation.

Wibulpolprasert S. 1999. Inequitable distribution of doctors: Can it be solved? *Human Resources for Health Development Journal* 3(1):2–39.

Wibulpolprasert S, Pengpaibon P. 2003. Integrated strategies to tackle inequitable distribution of doctors in Thailand: Four decades of experience. *Human Resources for Health* 1(1):12.

World Bank. 1993. *World Development Report 1993: Investing in Health*. New York, NY: Oxford University Press.

Wyss K. 2004. *Scaling Up Antiretroviral Treatment and Human Resources for Health: What Are the Challenges in sub-Saharan Africa?* Berne, Switzerland: Swiss Agency for Development and Cooperation.

2

Confronting HIV/AIDS on the Ground

Pandemic: A disease affecting the majority of the population of a large region, or which is epidemic in many different parts of the world (Thomas, 1973:P-12).

In the fourteenth century, the Black Death[1] ravaged Europe, killing a third of its population. In the sixteenth century, smallpox claimed the lives of approximately 17 million New World Indians and felled the great Aztec and Inca Empires. In the early twentieth century, influenza killed countless numbers in Europe, Asia, Australia, and the Americas—affecting one-quarter of the world's population. Throughout human history, epic infectious outbreaks have occurred periodically, leaving victims of all ages, races, and economic status in their wake. Today, however, the poor bear the brunt of epidemic infections, both acute and chronic. Exacerbated by a lingering burden of malnutrition, scant or absent health services, and other risk factors, malaria, tuberculosis (TB), vaccine-preventable diseases, and simple respiratory and diarrheal ailments continue to plague the world's neediest populations. Just a few decades ago, these diseases represented the primary unfinished agenda in global health.

That situation changed with the emergence of HIV/AIDS, the modern successor to the great pandemics of history. Twenty-five years after first being recognized in humans, the disease has now claimed more than 20

---

[1]A bacterial infection caused by *Yersinia pestis*, also known as the plague.

million lives, and close to 40 million people worldwide harbor HIV (UNAIDS, 2004). Of the latter, 30 million are Africans, concentrated in southern and eastern Africa where HIV prevalence among adults now exceeds 15 percent in many countries and 30 percent in at least four countries (Botswana, Lesotho, Swaziland, and Zimbabwe). In less than 10 years, HIV/AIDS has reversed the gains in life expectancy achieved by Africa over 50 years and orphaned 12 million children, half of whom are between the ages of 10 and 14 (UNAIDS, 2004). Girls and women are especially vulnerable to HIV, and now account for 50 percent of people living with HIV worldwide and 57 percent of those in sub-Saharan Africa (UNAIDS, 2004).

At the same time, HIV/AIDS increasingly threatens other regions of the world. According to the National Intelligence Council, by 2010 China will likely have 10–15 million people living with HIV, India 20–25 million, and Russia 5–8 million (Morrison, 2004).

Viewed from the perspective of the wreckage of human lives, there is nothing positive about HIV/AIDS. However, unlike earlier pandemics that took place in the absence of knowledge, tools, and connectivity, today's crisis offers one opportunity: a decisive global response. What form should this response take? Rich countries have a moral and political imperative to invest heavily in effective treatments and other material assistance to poor countries highly impacted by HIV/AIDS. Yet no amount of money can fully substitute for experienced professionals with a variety of skills assisting counterparts on the ground in fighting the epidemic.

This chapter begins by examining the linkages between HIV/AIDS and two other infectious diseases—TB and malaria—that have a major impact on the developing world, as well as the resulting health care challenges. This is followed by an overview of the impacts of HIV/AIDS at the individual, household, and societal levels. Next, the chapter provides a closer look at HIV/AIDS, itself, including its pathophysiology, transmission, and natural course, and comorbidities and cofactors in disease progression. Finally, the chapter reviews treatment and care for HIV/AIDS, addressing in turn antiretroviral therapy (ART), the problem of drug resistance, elements of a comprehensive care model for those infected in developing countries, clinical entry points for treatment and care, and issues in providing ART and HIV/AIDS care in resource-limited settings.

HIV/AIDS, TUBERCULOSIS, AND MALARIA

Linkages Among the Three Diseases

In an attempt to target high-risk individuals, health programs addressing malaria, TB, and HIV infection often focus on biologically vulnerable groups. Table 2-1 summarizes the available evidence on biological and

TABLE 2-1 Available Evidence on Biological and Disease-Related
Vulnerability Factors

Vulnerability Factor	Malaria	Tuberculosis	HIV/AIDS
Age	Children under 5, high endemicity; all ages, low endemicity	Children under 5 and adults	Young adults
Pregnancy	Strong evidence for association	Weak evidence for association	No evidence for association
Male/Female Ratio	Equal	Children, M=F; adults M>F	Adolescents M<F; adults M=F
Genetic Influences on Infection or Disease Vulnerability	Ethnic traits, red-cell abnormalities, HLA/MHC[a] markers	Ethnic traits, genes for vitamin D receptor	Chemokine receptors (for example, CCR5)
Interactions	Coinfection with HIV increases degree and severity of infection	Coinfection with HIV increases disease progression	Other sexually transmitted diseases increase HIV infectiousness

[a]HLA/MHC = human leukocyte antigen /major histocompatibility complex.
SOURCE: Adapted from Bates and colleagues (2004).
Reprinted, with permission, from Elsevier (*The Lancet Infectious Diseases* 2004:268).

disease-related vulnerability factors. Depending on the disease, infants, children under age 5, girls and women, pregnant women, and people of reproductive age are particularly vulnerable to infection.

While the approach of focusing on biologically vulnerable groups is useful in planning health interventions, poverty and a lack of education and available health services all contribute to the bigger picture (Bates et al., 2004). Indeed, the World Health Organization has identified the world's 1.2 billion people living in absolute poverty as most vulnerable to malaria, TB, and HIV infection (WHO, 2002b). High burdens of these diseases contribute to national and individual poverty, linking poverty and disease in a downward spiral. Moreover, low general educational attainment and a lack of knowledge about HIV transmission correlate with increased rates of risky behavior and HIV infection (Bates et al., 2004). HIV/AIDS and malaria also restrict opportunities for formal education: HIV/AIDS has caused reductions in school enrollment of up to 36 percent in some parts of Africa (Cohen, 1999), while malaria accounts for 10 to 50 percent of school days lost to illness in sub-Saharan Africa (Sachs and Malaney, 2002). Certain occupations or livelihoods also increase the risk of acquiring HIV (e.g., female sex workers, long-distance truck drivers), malaria (e.g., rural subsistence farmers, forest workers), and TB (e.g., workers exposed to silica and other dusts).

Medical linkages among the three diseases are fairly well established, with the evidence for a link between HIV/AIDS and TB being quite compelling. TB is a leading killer of people with HIV/AIDS, and up to 80 percent of TB patients are HIV positive in countries with a high prevalence of HIV (Ruxin et al., 2005). Although not as strong, an association between HIV infection and clinical malaria has also been identified in pregnant women (Ladner et al., 2002, 2003). Additionally, antimicrobial drug resistance and treatment delays complicate all three diseases, increasing transmission, morbidity, and mortality.

Given that these three diseases are the top infectious disease killers in the world today, and given the linkages described above, some believe that investing solely in combating one disease may compromise the building of local capacities to foster broader health benefits (Tan et al., 2003). The belief is that until systems are in place to deliver essential health services on a large scale, progress against one disease will be achieved at the price of neglecting others. It is thought that lasting control of HIV, TB, and malaria will depend on strengthening health systems as well as disease-specific programs (Ruxin et al., 2005).

Current Scope

As noted in Chapter 1, close to 40 million people are currently estimated to be living with HIV/AIDS, 95 percent of them in developing countries, particularly sub-Saharan Africa. In 2004 alone, almost 5 million people are thought to have become infected with HIV, including 2 million women and 800,000 children. The estimated total number of AIDS deaths in 2004 was 3.1 million (UNAIDS, 2004).

TB, a progressive and debilitating bacterial infection caused by *Mycobacterium tuberculosis* and spread from person to person by coughing and sneezing, is the world's second most common cause of death from infectious disease after HIV/AIDS, killing nearly 2 million people and causing 8 to 9 million new infections each year (Frieden et al., 2003). Of the 40 million people currently living with HIV/AIDS worldwide, one-third are coinfected with TB, most of these living in sub-Saharan Africa (WHO, 2002c). HIV/AIDS and TB are so closely connected that the term "coepidemic" or "dual epidemic" is used to describe their relationship.

Malaria, a parasitic infection transmitted by *Anopheles* mosquitoes, causes 1 to 2 million deaths worldwide every year, more than 90 percent of which are in sub-Saharan Africa among children under 5, although adults also suffer morbidity and mortality from the disease. Malaria also threatens at least 24 million pregnancies annually and causes low birth weight, a four-fold risk factor for increased infant mortality. Malaria's burden on health systems is immense: 30 percent of all outpatient visits and 20 to 50 percent of all hospital admissions in affected countries in Africa are attributable to the disease (WHO, 2003c). Malaria's contribution to poverty is seen at the household level and in slowed economic growth overall. Populations living in regions of high malaria transmission in 1965 had annual economic growth rates that were 1.3 percent lower than those of other countries over the period 1965-1990 (Sachs and Malaney, 2002).

Health Care Challenges

The critical lack of human health care resources in the scale-up of HIV/ AIDS treatment and care was the central driver for this study. Several recent reviews and human resource assessments have emphasized the growing HIV-related work burden (which is also characterized by clinical and organizational complexity) juxtaposed against poor basic health services and weak human resources. To some extent, similar issues apply to TB and malaria, whose acute management and long-term control are only slightly less demanding than is the case for HIV/AIDS. TB diagnosis requires, at a minimum, high-quality sputum microscopy, and current treatment guidelines for uncomplicated infections require that patients take four drugs under direct supervision for their first 2 months of treatment, followed by two drugs for another 4 to 7 months. Effective and sustainable malaria control involves activities ranging from vector control, to intermittent preventive treatment of high-risk individuals, to epidemic forecasting. These measures are especially difficult to implement in settings of decentralized health care and shortages of skilled personnel. Malaria treatment is also complicated by growing drug resistance in most endemic countries, a situation that has led to an increase in deaths from the disease over 10 to 20 years; nonetheless, failing drugs such as chloroquine remain in widespread use, especially in sub-Saharan Africa (IOM, 2004). In 2002, the World Health Organization recommended that governments rapidly adopt more effective first-line malaria treatments, in particular, artemisinin-based combination therapies that are currently in limited global supply. Treatment of severe and complicated malaria requires a range of technically sophisticated diagnostic, therapeutic, and supportive interventions, depending on available local resources.

The Starting Point for HIV/AIDS Care:
Prevention, Education, and Awareness

Although American health professionals are proficient in many biomedical interventions and tools that can now be applied to the care of HIV/AIDS patients in the PEPFAR focus countries, it is still critically important to acknowledge behavioral interventions as a means of stemming the global HIV/AIDS epidemic. Failure to expand access to HIV prevention while scaling up ART in developing countries could lead to a situation similar to that in the industrialized world, where HIV prevention was insufficiently emphasized as HIV treatment was expanded; the result was increases in risk behavior and infection rates (Global HIV Prevention Working Group, 2004). Experience in the few countries in which generalized epidemics have been substantially curtailed, albeit limited, suggests that adequately resourced, politically supported national prevention programs addressing the behavioral mediators of HIV can change the course of the global HIV/AIDS epidemic by averting millions of infections (Harrison and Steinberg, 2002).

The prevention message—communicated at HIV treatment sites and through mass campaigns focused especially on young people (who are not as likely as adults to visit medical settings)—needs to reach those at high risk of infection, those considered to be at low risk, and those already infected. An effective prevention plan encompasses a set of strategies that achieve maximum impact when pursued in combination (Global HIV Prevention Working Group, 2004):

- Behavior change programs to promote condom use, reduced numbers of partners, mutual monogamy, abstinence, and delayed initiation of sexual activity
- Prevention and treatment of sexually transmitted diseases
- HIV counseling and testing
- Harm reduction programs for injecting drug users
- Prevention of mother-to-child transmission
- Blood safety practices
- Infection control in health care settings
- Policy reforms to reduce the vulnerability of women and girls, and to ensure the legality and availability of proven HIV prevention strategies, such as use of condoms and clean syringes
- Prevention programs specifically designed for people living with HIV

IMPACTS OF HIV/AIDS

The social, economic, and political impacts of HIV/AIDS affect all levels of society, from individuals and households to businesses and governments.

Socioeconomic Impacts on Households

By any measure, the death of a relative or other loved one to HIV/AIDS is a devastating event. In addition to the trauma of this loss, however, households may suffer a precipitous decline in living standards due to the loss of income previously generated by the victim and increased household spending on health-related goods and services. HIV/AIDS also lowers household income when family members reallocate time previously devoted to work to caring for a sick relative. Funeral expenses are another financial burden.

HIV/AIDS also has socioeconomic impacts on children. Rising poverty in general limits children's access to education, which is intimately linked to the accumulation of human capital (Bell et al., 2004). As households lose income and reallocate resources, children are at greater risk of malnutrition. After a parent's death, members of the extended family frequently care for the victim's children. Results of surveys conducted in 10 countries of sub-Saharan Africa between 1992 and 2000 reveal that orphans tend to live in poorer households than nonorphans and to have lower school enrollment rates, even after controlling for household income (Case et al., 2004).

Socioeconomic Impacts on the Private and Public Sectors

Beyond households, the economic effects of HIV/AIDS multiply. As the disease takes a toll on workers in the private sector, rising production costs erode competitiveness and deter investments. Resulting declines in economic growth weaken the domestic tax base and decrease revenues. Within the public sector, as public servants fall ill and die, the efficiency of government agencies deteriorates. Further disruptions in public services occur when sick employees take extended leave or government agencies lag in hiring their replacements. The impacts of such disruptions are particularly severe for decentralized government services, such as local education and health care (Haacker, 2004).

The government sector most directly affected by HIV/AIDS is the health sector (Over, 2004). The demands on public health services rise sharply with the spread of the epidemic; at the same time, many health personnel are themselves infected (see Chapter 1). Prior to the availability of ART, the percentage of hospital beds occupied by HIV patients—ranging from 30 to 70 percent—indicated that HIV/AIDS was absorbing much of the existing capacity of health services in highly affected countries.

Military Conflict and HIV/AIDS

At present, Africa has more civil conflicts than any other region in the world. African peacekeeping troops have recently helped to stabilize Liberia,

Burundi, and the Democratic Republic of the Congo. Thus it is important that the Joint United Nations Programme on HIV/AIDS (UNAIDS) conservatively estimates that men serving in armies have an HIV infection rate two to five times higher than that of their civilian counterparts (UNICEF, 2003). The South African government, for example, refuses to deploy its HIV-positive troops as peacekeepers (currently, 17 to 22 percent of South Africa's defense force is HIV positive) (South Africa Department of Defense, 2002). The health and capacity of African soldiers and peacekeepers are of particular concern at a time when major powers are reluctant to engage further in peacekeeping operations in the region.

Armed forces also play a role in propagating the epidemic. Not only is rape a weapon of war, but some military personnel exploit vulnerable civilians (especially children and young people), promising money, food, or protection of shelter in exchange for sex. And when HIV-positive soldiers return home, they put their sexual partners at risk.

Finally, the breakdown of families and communities leaves children vulnerable to recruitment into armed groups. Two-thirds of the 300,000 children under age 18 involved in armed conflict worldwide are in Africa; many are under age 10 (Amnesty International, 2003). In addition to physical injury and disability, these children are at risk of sexually transmitted diseases, including HIV/AIDS (Uppard, 2003).

A CLOSER LOOK AT HIV/AIDS

HIV is a single-stranded ribonucleic acid (RNA) virus of the *Retroviridae* family. Following acquisition of HIV, individuals remain infected for life as a result of integration of the retroviral genome into the genome of various human cells. Without treatment, the virus causes a progressive weakening of the human immune system, eventually culminating in AIDS and death.

One of the major direct mechanisms by which HIV leads to illness is the selective infection and destruction of certain cells, known as CD4 lymphocytes or CD4 T-cells. This depletion in turn progressively disables an important component of the human immune system.

AIDS represents the most advanced stage of HIV infection, when severe complications occur; these include a variety of infections of the lungs, brain, eyes, and other organs, as well as debilitating weight loss, diarrhea, and certain cancers. The U.S. Centers for Disease Control and Prevention (CDC) has identified numerous opportunistic infections and cancers that, in the presence of HIV infection, constitute an AIDS diagnosis. In 1993, CDC expanded the criteria for an AIDS diagnosis in adults and adolescents to include a CD4 T-cell count at or below 200 cells per microliter in the presence of HIV infection (above the age of 5, persons with normally functioning immune systems usually have CD4 T-cell counts in the range of 500 to 1,500 cells per microliter).

Transmission

The three primary routes of HIV transmission are sexual contact; perinatal transmission from infected mothers to their infants; and exposure to blood through injection drug use, transfusion, and accidental exposure to blood-contaminated sharps and needle sticks.

Heterosexual transmission is the major mode of spread of HIV infection in Africa (Cohn et al., 2001). High rates of heterosexual transmission in Africa may be partly attributable to a higher prevalence of genital ulcer disease, since genital ulcers increase the infectiousness of both male and female source partners (Piot and Laga, 1989; Plummer et al., 1991). Nonulcerative sexually transmitted diseases, such as gonorrhea and chlamydial infection, also increase sexual transmission of HIV (Laga et al., 1993; Plummer et al., 1991). Even more important, the infectiousness of a source partner increases with advancing immunodeficiency, that is, lower CD4 T-cell counts and higher viral loads (Quinn et al., 2000).

Vertical transmission of HIV from an infected woman to her infant can occur during intrauterine gestation, delivery, or the postpartum period via breastfeeding. The burden of pediatric HIV infection is directly linked to HIV prevalence among pregnant women, which exceeds 25 percent in some parts of Africa. The risk of mother-to-child transmission also correlates with increasing immunosuppression and maternal viral load.

Finally, people who receive blood or blood products from HIV-infected donors are at very high risk for HIV infection. Among injecting drug users, HIV is transmitted by parenteral exposure to HIV-infected blood via contaminated needles and other injection equipment. Accidental percutaneous, mucous membrane, and cutaneous exposures to blood-contaminated body fluids can occur in any health care setting, but are most common in resource-limited settings, where education and personal protective equipment may be lacking.

Preventing Transmission

More than two decades of research has firmly established that certain interventions can reduce high-risk sexual and needle-sharing behaviors that lead to HIV infection (Coates and Szekeres, 2004). In the United States, sex education is considered a cornerstone of the prevention of HIV, other sexually transmitted diseases, and teenage pregnancy (Kirby, 2001). An analysis of the "ABC" (abstinence, be faithful, use condoms) prevention model in Uganda indicated that delaying intercourse, reducing the number of partners, and using condoms contributed to recently lowered HIV rates in that country (Stoneburner and Low-Beer, 2004). However, the ABC strategy fails to address some daunting problems. Chief among these is the fact that abstinence among young women in the face of sexual violence is difficult or impossible to ensure (Pettifor et al., 2004). A South African study found that women in violent relationships were 50 percent more likely to have HIV than their counterparts in nonviolent relationships (Dunkle et al., 2004). In addition, most young women in sub-Saharan Africa acquire HIV from steady partners or spouses (KIT et al., 1995).

As ART scale-up occurs in high-impact areas, voluntary testing and counseling will become increasingly prominent in comprehensive HIV/AIDS prevention strategies. The view that Africa should move swiftly toward widespread voluntary conseling and testing—especially for all patients admitted to hospitals or treated for TB—is gaining increasing support among medical experts and African leaders (DeCock et al., 2003; WHO, 2004). Brazil was the first country in the world to initiate universal voluntary counseling and testing, followed by Lesotho, whose HIV/AIDS prevalence rate of 30 percent is the fourth highest in the world. In Botswana (where HIV prevalence among adults stands at 38 percent), testing has been offered routinely in all public medical facilities, including antenatal clinics, since January 2004.

Natural History of Disease

The clinical spectrum of HIV infection ranges from asymptomatic carriage, to acute infection, to advanced immunodeficiency with opportunistic disease. Results of early retrospective studies of HIV-infected homosexual men in San Francisco suggested that the incubation period from acute HIV infection to development of AIDS is 9.8 years (Bacchetti and Moss, 1989). Other early studies led to estimates of the incubation period ranging from 6.5 to 13 years, with an average of 8–9 years.

As HIV-related immunosuppression progresses, the spectrum of illness seen among the infected in the developing world differs from that seen in HIV-infected residents of western countries. In Africa, for instance, people with early HIV infection are more likely to develop TB, bacterial pneumonia, or septicemia. AIDS itself is more often associated with "slim disease" or disseminated fungal infections than with the classic opportunistic infections of western countries.

Because of their immunologic immaturity, the progression of HIV/AIDS in infants and young children is accelerated following vertical transmission from HIV-infected mothers. Without treatment, most HIV-infected children in Africa die before their third birthday (Chakraborty, 2005).

Comorbidities and Cofactors in Disease Progression

Many individuals who are either at risk for or become infected with HIV are also malnourished and coinfected with other diseases (see the discussion above); some also suffer from substance abuse and mental illness. A full understanding of the negative synergy between these comorbidities and HIV is just beginning to emerge; however, many researchers have shown that opportunistic infections—especially TB—increase the risk of death (Seage et al., 2002; Whalen et al., 2000). Recent evidence has also shown that malaria temporarily increases HIV viral loads (Kublin et al., 2005), theoretically increasing HIV transmission 50 percent during periods of active illness (Whitworth and Hewitt, 2005). HIV also worsens malaria in pregnant women, who experience more complications, as well as an increased risk of adverse birth outcomes, when they are HIV coinfected (ter Kuile et al., 2004).

Both acute and chronic malnutrition also reduce immunity to and accelerate the progression of HIV/AIDS (Anabwani and Navario, 2005). At the macro level, bidirectional links exist between HIV/AIDS and food security within households and entire regions affected by acute famine (Griekspoor et al., 2004). Decreased availability of food also affects HIV/AIDS transmission by forcing people to adopt risky survival strategies, such as transactional sex.

TREATMENT AND CARE

Antiretroviral Therapy[2]

The goal of ART is to inhibit viral replication while minimizing the side effects and toxicities of currently used drugs. The inhibition of HIV replication permits restoration of the immune system. Although viral eradication from the host genome is not yet possible, appropriate lifelong administration of antiretrovirals (plus other drugs to prevent opportunistic infections), can reduce AIDS-related mortality to almost zero for the remainder of a patient's life, allowing the patient to enjoy an enhanced quality of life and remain productive.

The benefits of antiretrovirals may be clinically observed in many ways, but restoration of immune function and suppression of viral replication are best evaluated by laboratory testing. The goal of therapy is to achieve a CD4 cell count greater than 200 mm^3 and an "undetectable" viral load

---

[2]This section is largely drawn from IOM (2005).

(< 50 copies/ml). With an effective regimen, these goals should be achieved within 4–6 months of initiating ART and can be maintained indefinitely if the patient continues to take the drugs.

There are now more than 20 drugs used to treat HIV/AIDS, falling into four classes. The first three classes of drug, affecting viral enzymes, are the nucleoside analogue reverse transcriptase inhibitors (NRTIs, exemplified by the very first antiretroviral, zidovudine or AZT, introduced in 1987); the nonnucleoside reverse transcriptase inhibitors (NNRTIs); and protease inhibitors (PIs). The most recently developed class of drugs, fusion inhibitors, block the entry of HIV into host target cells such as CD4 lymphocytes. In addition to possessing separate mechanisms of action, each class also possesses unique effects and toxicities.[3]

Triple combinations are the most effective way to treat HIV infection. Highly active antiretroviral therapy (HAART) refers to a daily regimen of treatment involving three or more drugs from at least two of the above classes. Mono or dual therapy, used at the start of the epidemic, is less effective and is associated with regimen failure and drug resistance.

Specific guidelines for use of antiretrovirals change regularly as new drugs are approved and the drawbacks of older drugs become more apparent. A comprehensive reference on the use of antiretroviral agents in HIV-infected adults and adolescents was recently released by the U.S. Department Health and Human Services (DHHS, 2005), and regular updates are provided at the reference website. It should be noted, however, that these guidelines derive from clinical and translational research undertaken in the United States and Europe, and that questions regarding their applicability to resource-limited settings remain.[4] Although guidelines based on Western experience provide a good starting point for scaling up ART in resource-limited settings, ongoing research conducted in these settings will be critical to the guidelines' ultimate success.

---

[3]For example, different drugs within the NRTI class may produce lactic acidosis, fatty liver, peripheral nerve damage, inflammation of the pancreas, and anemia. Drugs within the NNRTI class often cause rash and liver function abnormalities. Drugs within the PI class may produce kidney stones and gastrointestinal side effects such as nausea and diarrhea. Combining antiretrovirals and TB treatment can also pose difficulties and require special monitoring.

[4]For example, in settings where patients' genetics and metabolic pathways differ from those of clinical trial populations, unexpected drug toxicities could develop. Moreover, different strains (clades) of virus circulate in Africa and Asia, raising questions about unexpected drug resistance patterns and the general applicability of drug sequencing algorithms developed in western countries. Finally, different opportunistic pathogens could change the clinical manifestations of HIV/AIDS in resource-limited settings and create new drug–drug interactions between antiretrovirals and specific treatments for opportunistic infections.

The Problem of Antiretroviral Resistance

Because HIV undergoes high rates of replication and turnover, its potential for developing drug resistance is great. It is currently believed that in the United States, 50 percent of patients receiving ART harbor a virus that is resistant to at least one antiretroviral drug (Richman et al., 2004). Resistance to a single drug or an entire class can develop during drug therapy (Clavel and Hance, 2004), or drug-resistant viral strains may be transmitted de novo to new hosts. One of the greatest concerns in scaling up ART in developing countries is the potential for drug resistance to develop and spread on a large scale, a situation that would ultimately jeopardize the treatment of all untreated populations exposed to high burdens of drug-resistant virus. The World Health Organization recommends that countries planning to implement ART programs concurrently introduce sentinel surveillance systems for HIV drug resistance.

The presence of a resistant virus in a population also complicates the delivery of ART at the local level because it necessitates diagnostic tests for resistance testing, the expertise to interpret and act upon the test results, and a larger armamentarium of antiretroviral drugs. These factors, in turn, increase the complexity and cost of treatment and make it difficult for midlevel practitioners to treat large populations.

While many factors can promote resistance to antiretroviral drugs in an individual patient,[5] the single most important safeguard against the development of drug resistance is adherence to the prescribed regimen. If at least 95 percent of doses are taken, there is a greater than 80 percent chance that the viral load will drop to less than 500 copies/ml; if fewer than 95 percent of doses are taken, fewer than 50 percent of patients achieve this level of viral suppression (Bartlett, 2004). Any regimen that does not completely suppress viral replication will eventually lead to drug resistance.

Treatment and Prevention of Opportunistic Infections

When the immune system of an HIV-infected individual is depleted to the point of AIDS, patients develop a range of secondary opportunistic infections such as TB; *Pneumocystis* pneumonia; cryptococcal meningitis; *Toxoplasma* brain abscesses; and HIV-related cancers, including Kaposi's sarcoma and lymphoma.

---

[5]Examples of such factors include the improper prescription of antiretrovirals; underdosing, leading to suboptimal drug levels; poor adherence to medication; missed doses of one or more drugs due to local stock-outs; altered drug metabolism; and the presence of tissue "sanctuaries" where virions evade the action of specific drugs.

Although potent combination antiretroviral treatments have reduced the incidence of opportunistic infections for many HIV-infected patients in developed countries, such infections remain a prominent feature of later stages of HIV infection and the common AIDS-defining events. A recent report published by CDC, the National Institutes of Health, and the HIV Medicine Association/Infectious Diseases Society of America lists treatment recommendations for 28 opportunistic infections due to protozoa, bacteria, fungi, and (nonretroviral) viruses in HIV-infected adults and adolescents (Benson et al., 2004).

Strategies for prevention of opportunistic infections in developing countries have not yet been fully developed. When available and tolerated, however trimethoprim-sulfamethoxazole (a broad-spectrum antibiotic) given to patients with CD4 cell counts below 200 mm^3 is generally accepted as a highly beneficial complement to ART (personal communication, Robert Schooley, University of California-San Francisco, February 14, 2005).

Comprehensive Health Care for HIV/AIDS in Developing Countries

Ideally, a comprehensive approach to treatment and care for people with HIV/AIDS includes a range of components, including the following:

- Community and national treatment, care, and prevention guidelines
- Education and awareness programs
- Programs to address stigma and discrimination
- Voluntary counseling and testing with informed consent in health facilities, along with services targeting vulnerable and difficult-to-reach populations
- Prevention of mother-to-child transmission
- Prevention and treatment of opportunistic and sexually transmitted infections
- Antiretroviral therapy and monitoring, including essential laboratory and clinical backup and drug management systems
- Embedded operations research programs designed to elucidate the most effective approaches to HIV/AIDS care and delivery in resource-limited settings
- Adherence support
- Social protection, nutrition, and welfare and psychosocial services
- Palliative and home-based care
- Bereavement support

In reality, however, different models of comprehensive health care delivery for HIV/AIDS will be needed to respond to the diverse requirements and capacities of the developing countries in which the infection is endemic. The introduction of treatment and care should also be appropriately phased. For example, ART should be initiated only if certain minimum conditions are met, including community preparedness, counseling and testing with informed consent, training of personnel for provision of ART and follow-up, and uninterrupted supplies of antiretroviral drugs. One key element is the training, support, accreditation, and quality control of providers, including those in both the public and private sectors (WHO, 2003a).

Another priority is reliable and confidential systems for medical record keeping (in some cases, such systems will be introduced into health facilities with no previous experience with using written medical records). Some countries are planning to use traditional paper-based systems combined with patient identity or photo cards. Others are exploring the potential use of new technologies, such as "smart cards" or fingerprint readers, barcoded drug packaging, and electronic databases for patient and drug monitoring. In Brazil, for example, most patients now receive a magnetic card, which they present to receive treatment (Attawell and Mundy, 2003).

Finally, caregiving and palliative measures—generally defined as pain and symptom management, advance care planning, prioritization of life goals, and support for individuals and families throughout the course of disease—will be essential elements of any comprehensive treatment program. This is a pressing need in Asia (Coughlan, 2003) as well as in Africa, a continent currently experiencing, in the words of one local hospice educator, "an epidemic of death" (Ramsay, 2003:1813). One survey of 48 African palliative care services for patients with AIDS found that 94 percent had experienced obstacles, especially a lack of trained providers; stigma; and government restrictions limiting access to narcotics such as oral morphine, which controls pain and diarrhea in the terminal phases of AIDS and allows many patients to stay in their homes without the cost or disruption of transfer to a hospital (Harding et al., 2003). Research from Uganda also suggests that dying patients' greatest need is relief of pain and other terminal symptoms (Kikule, 2003).

Uganda is the first and only African country thus far to make palliative care for people in the terminal stages of AIDS and cancer part of its national health plan (Ramsay, 2003). Although only a small number of eligible Ugandans are currently accessing palliative care and free oral morphine, the government is revising its laws to enable wider prescribing by community nurse specialists. The need for better community-based palliative and end-of-life models in many low-resource settings heavily impacted by HIV/AIDS is reflected in the fact that 15 percent of PEPFAR funds in target countries is allocated to palliative care initiatives.

Entry Points for HIV/AIDS Treatment and Care in Developing Countries

Experience with pilot programs has revealed several ways to integrate prevention and care efforts through various clinical entry points, including voluntary counseling and testing, sexual and reproductive health services, and other health services.

Voluntary Counseling and Testing

Voluntary counseling and testing with informed consent is the key point at which people learn their HIV status and are offered care services, as well as behavioral and preventive advice. Studies have shown that voluntary counseling and testing consistently increases safe-sex behaviors among people who are HIV positive (CDC, 2000; Weinhardt et al., 1999), as well as those who are HIV negative (Spielberg et al., 2003; The Voluntary HIV-1 Counseling and Testing Efficacy Study Group, 2000).

Until recently, however, access to voluntary counseling and testing in countries most severely affected by HIV/AIDS has been limited. As a result, there are few developing countries in which more than 10 percent of the adult population has been tested (Fylkesnes and Siziya, 2004). Greater provision of HIV treatment should create greater demand for counseling and testing services (MSF South Africa et al., 2003; Mukherjee et al., 2003). The increasing need for such services in developing countries—reaching geographically remote areas as well as community clinics and networks—must parallel the scale-up of other HIV-related services. Otherwise, limited availability of testing and counseling could become a bottleneck to expanded treatment and care. The actual training of providers in voluntary counseling and testing takes 1 to 8 weeks (Heiby, 2004).

Rapid testing methods that can provide reliable results within minutes and require relatively little laboratory capacity are a practical tool for voluntary counseling and testing outreach settings in developing countries. More than 60 rapid tests have been developed and used overseas (Cohen et al., 2003). For confirmation of HIV status, a two-step rapid testing strategy may be more cost-effective than the standard combination of enzyme immunoassay followed by a confirmatory Western blot used in most Western countries (Ekwueme et al., 2003).

UNAIDS has identified several critical elements of counseling and testing programs: testing should be voluntary, results should be confidential, testing should focus on an individual client's needs, HIV-positive and HIV-negative persons should be referred for ongoing support, and stigma-reducing activities should be incorporated into the services provided (CDC, 2004; UNAIDS, 2000). Unfortunately, anticipated and actual stigma directed at HIV-infected individuals still constrains the use of testing services

(Parker and Aggleton, 2003). HIV-infected women who disclose their status are also vulnerable to partner violence and economic instability (Mamam et al., 2000, 2002).

Sexual and Reproductive Health Services

Sexual and reproductive health services, including clinics for treatment of other sexually transmitted infections, are another entry point for HIV/AIDS prevention and care. Antenatal services provide access to programs to prevent mother-to-child transmission of HIV and allow HIV-infected women to receive treatment and care during and after pregnancy, as well as advice for future pregnancies (WHO, 2003b). Outreach services for targeted populations, including sex workers, men who have sex with men, and injecting drug users are further channels for information.

Routine testing of pregnant women (with the right to refuse) is recommended as part of worldwide efforts to expand access to ART and programs to prevent mother-to-child transmission of HIV, in the 2004 joint United Nations and World Health Organization policy statement on HIV testing (UNAIDS Global Reference Group on HIV/AIDS and Human Rights, 2004). Without intervention, 35 to 40 percent of HIV-positive women transmit HIV to their infants. With drug prophylaxis and formula feeding, transmission is reduced to 5 to 10 percent, and with combination ART, transmission falls below 1 percent (Nolan et al., 2002). The consensus of the international public health community is to recommend the unrestricted use of any of the short-course antiretroviral regimens of validated efficacy for prevention of mother-to-child transmission, especially in areas of high HIV prevalence (UNAIDS, 1999).

Other Health Services

Other health services, in particular TB programs, have the potential to recruit large numbers of people into HIV treatment. As the TB and HIV/AIDS epidemics continue to fuel each other, increased collaboration between programs is essential. It has also been proposed that TB programs assist in the delivery of ART and HIV prevention services. For example, the Haiti Partners in Health Program has found that the directly observed therapy short course (DOTS) approach used for TB treatment can be equally effective for ART (Farmer et al., 2001). Others argue, however, that DOTS and ART strategies are not readily interchangeable, since TB treatment is time limited, while ART is lifelong. Concerns also exist regarding the risk of cross-infection in TB treatment facilities if HIV-infected individuals come into frequent contact with contagious TB patients.

The World Health Organization's Strategy for Chronic Disease Care in Developing Countries

Although HIV infection has dramatically lowered life expectancy in much of sub-Saharan Africa, life expectancy in many developing countries has continued to increase over the past decade. Chronic conditions such as diabetes and cardiovascular disease now account for roughly half of all health services required in the developing world (WHO, 2002a). To address these new trends in human health, the World Health Organization recently proposed a global strategy for designing and reconfiguring health care systems to better meet the needs of people with chronic diseases (see Box 2-1). This strategy could serve as a model for delivering comprehensive services to HIV-infected people. The approach starts with education and voluntary counseling and testing, followed by the initiation of ART and prevention of opportunistic infections, and culminating in the medical management of advanced HIV/AIDS by progressively tiered health professionals.

BOX 2-1
The World Health Organization's Strategy for Comprehensive Chronic Disease Care in the Developing World

- Shift the emphasis from acute, episodic care to providing continuity of care with planned visits and regular follow-up.
- Develop health policies, collaboration, legislation, and health care financing to support comprehensive care strategies.
- Emphasize delivery of services at the primary care level to ensure the broadest access to effective care.
- Develop effective communication and referral systems among the primary, secondary, and tertiary levels of health care.
- Center care on the patient, educate patients about their disease so they can become active participants in their care, and promote adherence to long-term treatment regimens.
- Link care to community resources; provide education and support to family and community members to assist in care.
- Emphasize prevention.
- Monitor and evaluate the quality of services and long term patient outcomes.

SOURCE: Kitahata et al. (2002).

Issues in Providing Antiretroviral Therapy and HIV/AIDS Care in Resource-Limited Settings

Many lessons are being learned in the early stages of providing ART in resource-limited settings. Among these is identification of the following needs: to strengthen health care systems; to define adequate infrastructure encompassing clinical care, laboratory, and pharmacy facilities for the delivery of ART; to overcome chronic shortages of staff at all levels of clinical care facilities; and to rethink training strategies and methods while incorporating continuing education, given the rapidly evolving nature of ART (Attawell and Mundy, 2003).

Although a detailed discussion of challenges and solutions is beyond the scope of this report, innovative programs will continue to serve as international demonstrations of treatment and care approaches. At the same time, many medically eligible patients will not have access to ART over the next few years because of financial or other constraints. Socioeconomic, geographic (rural versus urban), and gender criteria for determining which patients will receive free or subsidized ART need to be carefully defined to ensure equitable access. It has been argued that governments that make deliberate choices about rationing ART and then explain and defend those choices are more likely to sustain economic development and social cohesion over the course of the epidemic than those that avoid the public policy debate and otherwise skirt decision making about equitable access to ART and other forms of HIV/AIDS care (Rosen et al., 2005).

REFERENCES

Amnesty International. 2003. *War: A Child's Game*. [Online]. Available: http://web.amnesty.org/pages/childsoldiers-index-eng [accessed March 1, 2005].

Anabwani G, Navario P. 2005. Nutrition and HIV/AIDS in sub-Saharan Africa: An overview. *Nutrition* 21(1):96–99.

Attawell K, Mundy J. 2003. *Provision of Antiretroviral Therapy in Resource-Limited Settings: A Review of Experience up to August 2003*. [Online]. Available: http://www.who.int/3by5/publications/documents/dfid/en/ [accessed March 1, 2005].

Bacchetti P, Moss AR. 1989. Incubation period of AIDS in San Francisco. *Nature* 338(6212): 251–253.

Bartlett J. 2004. Antiretroviral treatment. In: *Infectious Diseases*. 3rd ed. Philadelphia, PA: Lippincott, Williams & Wilkins. Pp. 1028–1038.

Bates I, Fenton C, Gruber J, Lalloo D, Medina Lara A, Squire SB, Theobald S, Thomson R, Tolhurst R. 2004. Vulnerability to malaria, tuberculosis, and HIV/AIDS infection and disease. Part 1: Determinants operating at individual and household level. *Lancet Infectious Diseases* 4(5):267–277.

Bell C, Davarajan S, Gersbach H. 2004. Thinking about the long-run economic costs of AIDS. In: Haacker M, ed. *The Macroeconomics of HIV/AIDS*. Washington, DC: International Monetary Fund. Pp. 96–133. [Online]. Available: http://www.imf.org/external/pubs/ft/AIDS/eng/ [accessed March 1, 2005].

Benson C, Kaplan JE, Mansur H, Pau A, Holmes K. 2004. Treating opportunistic infections among HIV-infected adults and adolescents. *Morbidity and Mortality Weekly Report* 53(RR15):1–112.

Case A, Paxson C, Ableinger J. 2004. Orphans in Africa: Parental death, poverty, and school enrollment. *Demography* 41:483–508.

CDC (Centers for Disease Control and Prevention). 2000. Adoption of protective behaviors among persons with recent HIV infection and diagnosis: Alabama, New Jersey, and Tennessee, 1997–1998. *Morbidity and Mortality Weekly Report* 49(23):512–515.

CDC. 2004. *Global AIDS Program: Strategy on Voluntary Counseling and Testing (VCT).* [Online]. Available: http://www.cdc.gov/nchstp/od/gap/pa_hiv.htm [accessed March 1, 2005].

Chakraborty R. 2005. HIV-1 infection in children: A clinical and immunologic overview. *Current HIV Research* 3(1):31–41.

Clavel F, Hance AJ. 2004. HIV drug resistance. *New England Journal of Medicine* 350(10): 1023–1035.

Coates TJ, Szekeres G. 2004. A Plan for the next generation of HIV prevention research: Seven key policy investigative challenges. *American Psychologist* 59(8):747–757.

Cohen D. 1999. *The HIV Epidemic and the Education Sector in sub-Saharan Africa: UNDP.* Issues Paper 32. [Online]. Available: http://www.undp.org/hiv/publications/issues/english/issue32e.htm [accessed March 1, 2005].

Cohen MH, Olszewski Y, Branson B, Robey M, Love F, Jamieson DJ, Bulterys M. 2003. Using point-of-care testing to make rapid HIV-1 tests in labor really rapid. *AIDS* 17(14): 2121–2124.

Cohn M, Frankel SS, Rugpao S, Young M, Willet G, Tovanabutra S, Khamboonruang C, VanCott T, Bhoopat L, Barrick S, Fox C, Quinn T, Vahey M, Nelson K, Weissman D. 2001. Chronic inflammation with increased human immunodeficiency virus (HIV) RNA expression in the vaginal epithelium of HIV-infected Thai women. *Journal of Infectious Diseases* 184(4):410–417.

Coughlan M. 2003. Pain and palliative care for people living with HIV/AIDS in Asia. *Journal of Pain & Palliative Care Pharmacotherapy* 17(3–4):91–104; discussion 105–106.

DeCock KM, Marum E, Mbori-Ngacha D. 2003. A serostatus-based approach to HIV/AIDS prevention and care in Africa. *Lancet* 362(9398):1847–1849.

DHHS (Department of Health and Human Services). 2005. *AIDSinfo Antiretroviral Treatment Adult and Adolescent Guidelines.* [Online]. Available: http://aidsinfo.nih.gov/guidelines/default_db2.asp?id=50 [accessed April 27, 2005].

Dunkle KL, Jewkes RK, Brown HC, Gray GE, McIntryre JA, Harlow SD. 2004. Gender-based violence, relationship power, and risk of HIV infection in women attending antenatal clinics in South Africa. *Lancet* 363(9419):1415–1421.

Ekwueme DU, Pinkerton SD, Holtgrave DR, Branson BM. 2003. Cost comparison of three HIV counseling and testing technologies. *American Journal of Preventive Medicine* 25(2):112–121.

Farmer P, Leandre F, Mukherjee JS, Claude M, Nevil P, Smith-Fawzi MC, Koenig SP, Castro A, Becerra MC, Sachs J, Attaran A, Kim JY. 2001. Community-based approaches to HIV treatment in resource-poor settings. *Lancet* 358(9279):404–409.

Frieden TR, Sterling TR, Munsiff SS, Watt CJ, Dye C. 2003. Tuberculosis. *Lancet* 362(9387):887–899.

Fylkesnes K, Siziya S. 2004. A randomized trial on acceptability of voluntary HIV counselling and testing. *Tropical Medicine & International Health* 9(5):566–572.

Global HIV Prevention Working Group. 2004. *HIV Prevention in the Era of Expanded Treatment Access.* Kaiser Family Foundation and Bill and Melinda Gates Foundation. [Online]. Available: http://www.kff.org/hivaids/loader.cfm?url=/commonspot/security/getfile.cfm&PageID=36967 [accessed March 18, 2005].

Griekspoor A, Spiegel P, Aldis W, Harvey P. 2004. The health sector gap in the southern Africa crisis in 2002/2003. *Disasters* 28(4):388–404.

Haacker M. 2004. HIV/AIDS: The impact on the social fabric and the economy In: Haacker M, ed. *The Macroeconomics of HIV/AIDS*. Washington, DC: International Monetary Fund. Pp. 41–95. [Online]. Available: http://www.imf.org/external/pubs/ft/AIDS/eng/ [accessed March 1, 2005].

Harding R, Stewart K, Marconi K, O'Neill JF, Higginson IJ. 2003. Current HIV/AIDS end-of-life care in sub-Saharan Africa: A survey of models, services, challenges and priorities. *Biomed Central Public Health* 3(1):33.

Harrison D, Steinberg M. 2002. *Behaviour Change: The Cornerstone of HIV Prevention*. South Africa: LoveLife.

Heiby J. 2004 (December 1). *Quality of Care and Human Resources in HIV Healthcare Programs*. Presentation at the December 1, 2004 Workshop of the IOM Committee on Options for the Overseas Placement of U.S. Health Professionals, Washington, DC.

IOM (Institute of Medicine). 2004. *Saving Lives, Buying Time: Economics of Malaria Drugs in an Age of Resistance*. Arrow J, Panosian C, Gelband H, eds. Washington, DC: The National Academies Press.

IOM. 2005. *Scaling Up Treatment for the Global AIDS Pandemic: Challenges and Opportunities*. Washington, DC: The National Academies Press.

Kikule E. 2003. A good death in Uganda: Survey of needs for palliative care for terminally ill people in urban areas. *British Medical Journal* 327(7408):192–194.

Kirby D. 2001. *Emerging Answers: Research Findings on Programs to Reduce Teenage Pregnancy*. Washington, DC: National Campaign to Prevent Teen Pregnancy.

KIT (Royal Tropical Institute), SafAIDS (Southern Africa AIDS Information Dissemination Service), WHO (World Health Organization). 1995. *Facing the Challenges of HIV/AIDS/STDs: A Gender-based Response*. Amsterdam, the Netherlands: KIT Publishers.

Kitahata MM, Tegger MK, Wagner EH, Holmes KK. 2002. Comprehensive health care for people infected with HIV in developing countries. *British Medical Journal* 325:954–957.

Kublin JG, Patnaik P, Jere CS, Miller WC, Hoffman IF, Chimbiya N, Pendame R, Taylor TE, Molyneux ME. 2005. Effect of *Plasmodium falciparum* malaria on concentration of HIV-1-RNA in the blood of adults in rural Malawi: A prospective cohort study. *Lancet* 365(9455):233–240.

Ladner J, Leroy V, Simonon A, Karita E, Bogaerts J, de Clercq A, Van de Perre P, Dabis F. 2002. HIV infection, malaria, and pregnancy: A prospective cohort study in Kigali, Rwanda. *American Journal of Tropical Medicine and Hygiene* 66(1):56–60.

Ladner J, Leroy V, Karita E, Van de Perre P, Dabis F. 2003. Malaria, HIV, and pregnancy. *AIDS* 17(2):275–276.

Laga M, Monoka A, Kivuvu M, Malele B, Tuliza M, Nzila N, Goeman J, Behets F, Batter V, Alary M. 1993. Non-ulcerative sexually transmitted diseases as risk factors for HIV-1 transmission in women: Results from a cohort study. *AIDS* 7(1):95–102.

Maman S, Campbell J, Sweat MD, Gielen AC. 2000. The intersections of HIV and violence: Directions for future research and interventions. *Social Science & Medicine* 50(4):459–478.

Maman S, Mbwambo JK, Hogan NM, Kilonzo GP, Campbell JC, Weiss E, Sweat MD. 2002. HIV-positive women report more lifetime partner violence: Findings from a voluntary counseling and testing clinic in Dar es Salaam, Tanzania. *American Journal of Public Health* 92(8):1331–1337.

Morrison JS. 2004. *HIV/AIDS Pandemic and U.S. Leadership*. [Online]. Available: http://www.aspeninstitute.org/admin/index.asp?downloadid=1229 [accessed March 1, 2005].

MSF (Médecins sans Frontières) South Africa, the Department of Public Health at the University of Cape Town, and the Provincial Administration of the Western Cape, South Africa. 2003. *Antiretroviral Therapy in Primary Health Care: Experience of the Khayelitsha Programme in South Africa: A Case Study.* Geneva, Switzerland: WHO. [Online]. Available: http://www.who.int/hiv/pub/prev_care/en/South_Africa_E.pdf [accessed March 1, 2005].

Mukherjee J, Colas M, Farmer P, Léandre F, Lambert W, Raymonville M, Koenig S, Walton D, Névil P, Louissant N, Orélus C. 2003. *Access to Antiretroviral Treatment and Care: The Experience of the HIV Equality Initiative, Cange, Haiti: A Case Study.* Perspectives and Practice in Antiretroviral Treatment. Geneva, Switzerland: WHO.

Nolan ML, Greenberg AE, Fowler MG. 2002. A review of clinical trials to prevent mother-to-child HIV-1 transmission in Africa and inform rational intervention strategies. *AIDS* 6(15):1991–1999.

Over M. 2004. HIV/AIDS: The impact on the social fabric and the economy. In: Haacker M, ed. *The Macroeconomics of HIV/AIDS.* Washington, DC: International Monetary Fund. Pp. 311–344. [Online]. Available: http://www.imf.org/external/pubs/ft/AIDS/eng/ [accessed March 1, 2005].

Parker R, Aggleton P. 2003. HIV and AIDS-related stigma and discrimination: A conceptual framework and implications for action. *Social Science & Medicine* 57(1):13–24.

Pettifor AE, Rees HV, Steffenson A, Hlongwa-Madikizela L, MacPhail C, Vermaak K, Kleinschmidt I. 2004. *HIV and Sexual Behavior among Young South Africans: A National Survey of 15–24 Year Olds.* Johannesburg, South Africa: Reproductive Health Research Unit, University of the Witwatersrand.

Piot P, Laga M. 1989. Genital ulcers, other sexually transmitted diseases, and the sexual transmission of HIV. *British Medical Journal* 298(6674):623–624.

Plummer FA, Simonsen JN, Cameron DW, Ndinya-Achola JO, Kreiss JK, Gakinya MN, Waiyaki P, Cheang M, Piot P, Ronald AR. 1991. Cofactors in male–female sexual transmission of human immunodeficiency virus type 1. *Journal of Infectious Diseases* 163(2):233–239.

Quinn TC, Wawer MJ, Sewankambo N, Serwadda D, Li C, Wabwire-Mangen F, Meehan MO, Lutalo T, Gray RH. 2000. Viral load and heterosexual transmission of human immunodeficiency virus type 1. Rakai Project Study Group. *New England Journal of Medicine* 342(13):921–929.

Ramsay S. 2003. Leading the way in African home-based palliative care. Free oral morphine has allowed expansion of model home-based palliative care in Uganda. *Lancet* 362(9398):1812–1813.

Richman DD, Morton SC, Wrin T, Hellmann N, Berry S, Shapiro MF, Bozzette SA. 2004. The prevalence of antiretroviral drug resistance in the United States. *AIDS* 18(10):1393–1401.

Rosen S, Sanne I, Collier A, Simon JL. 2005. Hard choices: Rationing antiretroviral therapy for HIV/AIDS in Africa. *Lancet* 365(9456):354–356.

Ruxen J, Paluzzi J, Wilson P, Tozan Y, Kruk M, Teklehaimanot A. 2005. Emerging consensus in HIV/AIDS, malaria, tuberculosis, and access to essential medicines. *Lancet* 365: 618–621.

Sachs J, Malaney P. 2002. The economic and social burden of malaria. *Nature* 415(6872): 680–685.

Seage GR III, Losina E, Goldie SJ, Paltiel AD, Kimmel AD, Freedberg KA. 2002. The relationship of preventable opportunistic infections, HIV-1 RNA, and CD4 Cell counts to chronic mortality. *Journal of Acquired Immune Deficiency Syndromes* 30(4):421–428.

South Africa Department of Defense. 2002. *Current Status of the HIV Epidemic in the SA National Defense Force.* [Online]. Available: http://www.mil.za/CSANDF/ SurgeonGeneral/AIDSCampaign/MasiWeb2/index.htm [accessed March 1, 2005].

Spielberg F, Camp S, Ramachandra E. 2003 (July 27–30). *HIV Home Self-Testing: Can It Work?* (Abstract M1-A0101) Presented at the July 27–30, 2003, National HIV Prevention Conference, Atlanta, GA.

Stoneburner RL, Low-Beer D. 2004. Population-level HIV declines and behavioral risk avoidance in Uganda. [erratum appears in *Science* 2004, Vol. 306(5701):1477]. *Science* 304(5671):714–718.

Tan D, Upshur R, Ford N. 2003. Global plagues and the Global Fund: Challenges in the fight against HIV, TB and malaria. *BMC International Health and Human Rights* 3:2.

ter Kuile FO, Parise ME, Verhoeff FH, Udhayakumar V, Newman RD, van Eijk AM, Rogerson SJ, Steketee RW. 2004. The burden of co-infection with human immunodeficiency virus type 1 and malaria in pregnant women in sub-saharan Africa. *American Journal of Tropical Medicine & Hygiene* 71(2 Suppl):41–54.

The Voluntary HIV-1 Counseling and Testing Efficacy Study Group. 2000. Efficacy of voluntary HIV-1 counseling and testing in individuals and couples in Kenya, Tanzania, and Trinidad: A randomized trial. *Lancet* 356(9224):103–112.

Thomas C, ed. 1973. *Taber's Cyclopedic Medical Dictionary.* Philadelphia, PA: F.A. Davis Company. Pp. P-12.

UNAIDS (Joint United Nations Programme on HIV/AIDS). 1999. *Prevention of HIV Transmission from Mother to Child: Strategic Options.* Geneva, Switzerland: WHO.

UNAIDS. 2000. *Voluntary Counseling and Testing (VCT): UNAIDS Technical Update.* Geneva, Switzerland: WHO. [Online]. Available: http://www.emro.who.int/asd/ backgrounddocuments/egy0703/VCTTechnicalUpdate.pdf [accessed March 4, 2005].

UNAIDS. 2004. *2004 Report on the Global AIDS Epidemic: 4th Global Report.* Geneva, Switzerland: UNAIDS.

UNAIDS Global Reference Group on HIV/AIDS and Human Rights. 2004. *UNAIDS/WHO Policy Statement on HIV Testing.* Geneva, Switzerland: WHO. [Online]. Available: http:/ /www.who.int/hiv/pub/vct/en/hivtestingpolicy04.pdf [accessed March 1, 2005].

UNICEF (United Nations Children Fund). 2003. *Children, Armed Conflict and HIV/AIDS.* New York, NY: UNICEF. [Online]. Available: http://www.unicef.org/publications/files/ Children_Armed_Conflict_and_HIV_AIDS.pdf [accessed March 4, 2005].

Uppard S. 2003. Child soldiers and children associated with the fighting forces. *Medicine, Conflict and Survival* 19(2):121–127.

Weinhardt LS, Carey MP, Johnson BT, Bickham NL. 1999. Effects of HIV counseling and testing on sexual risk behavior: A meta-analytic review of published research, 1985–1997. *American Journal of Public Health* 89(9):1397–1405.

Whalen CC, Nsubuga P, Okwera A, Johnson JL, Hom DL, Michael NL, Mugerwa RD, Ellner JJ. 2000. Impact of pulmonary tuberculosis on survival of HIV-infected adults: A prospective epidemiologic study in Uganda. *AIDS* 14(9):1219–1228.

Whitworth JA, Hewitt KA. 2005. Effect of malaria on HIV-1 progression and transmission. *Lancet* 365(9455):196–197.

WHO (World Health Organization). 2002a. *Innovative Care for Chronic Conditions: Building Blocks for Action.* Geneva, Switzerland: WHO.

WHO. 2002b. *Scaling Up the Response to Infectious Diseases: A Way Out of Poverty.* Geneva, Switzerland: WHO.

WHO. 2002c. *Strategic Framework to Decrease the Burden of TB/HIV.* Geneva, Switzerland: WHO.

WHO. 2003a. *Emergency Scale-Up of Antiretroviral Therapy in Resource Limited Settings: Technical and Operational Recommendations to Achieve 3 by 5; Report of the WHO/UNAIDS International Congress Meeting on Technical and Operational Recommendations for Emergency Scaling-Up of Antiretroviral Therapy in Resource-Limited Settings.* Lusaka, Zambia, November 18–21, 2003.

WHO. 2003b. *Strategic Approaches to the Prevention of HIV Infections in Infants; Report of a WHO Meeting, Morges, Switzerland, March 20–22, 2002.* Geneva, Switzerland: WHO.

WHO. 2003c. *Africa Malaria Report.* Geneva, Switzerland: WHO.

WHO. 2004. *WHO Applauds Lesotho Prime Minister for Leading Universal Voluntary HIV Testing Drive.* [Online]. Available: http://www.who.int/3by5/newsitem6/en/print.html [accessed March 1, 2005].

3

New Routes of Engagement Against
Global HIV/AIDS

Much has been written about the early meager response to global HIV/AIDS on the part of governments, donor countries, and multinational institutions. The words of one medical author typify the feelings of many:

> Governments of severely affected nations have failed to provide leadership and national resources for HIV/AIDS prevention and care; donor countries have failed to increase levels of spending as the pandemic has escalated; and multinational lending and aid institutions have responded with bureaucratic lethargy and loans instead of grants. Moreover, the well-documented debate among public health experts on the relative merits and shortcomings of prevention versus [antiretroviral] management likely served to obfuscate priorities in donor and recipient governments. An additional source of consternation has been the exorbitant prices of [antiretroviral] medications for African countries (Anabwani and Navario, 2005:96–97).

In actuality, the last 3 years has witnessed dramatic breakthroughs in global HIV/AIDS assistance and control efforts: a sharp drop in the price of antiretroviral drugs, simplified drug delivery, greater political commitment among leaders in donor and recipient governments, greater involvement of the private sector, and major international initiatives. Total global spending on HIV/AIDS in low- and middle-income countries increased 500 percent between 1996 and 2003, reaching $4.7 billion in 2004 (UNAIDS, 2003), with 56 percent of this total going to Africa (IRINnews, 2004). On January 25, 2005, the U.S. Food and Drug Administration announced the tentative approval of the first generic, copackaged antiretroviral drug regimen (lamivudine/zidovudine and nevirapine, manufactured by Aspen

Pharmacare of South Africa) for use in the PEPFAR initiative. Whereas a mass scale-up of antiretroviral therapy (ART) was once considered unaffordable and technically unworkable, donors viewing the demography of the pandemic now view such a scale-up as possible if not essential, making it the centerpiece of several new initiatives.

At the same time, however, there are daunting barriers to implementing new HIV/AIDS programs and scaled up treatment in highly affected areas. These include a lack of trained and skilled personnel on the ground; ministries resisting urgent action; and the growing burden placed on highly affected countries by proliferating donor demands for comprehensive planning, reporting, monitoring, and evaluation. For many African countries that still spend less than $10 per capita per year on health, the provision of ART far exceeds national capacities; many countries also remain uneasy over donors' long-term commitment to (in most cases) still-growing populations of HIV-infected individuals (Morrison, 2004).

This chapter summarizes the history, funding, and targets of the United States' major international HIV/AIDS initiative (PEPFAR), as well as the World Health Organization's (WHO) 3 × 5 initiative and the United Nations (UN) Global Fund to Fight AIDS, Tuberculosis, and Malaria (Global Fund). The chapter also briefly summarizes other federal and research-based initiatives, and the efforts of major foundations and private-sector partners actively engaged in the international fight against HIV/AIDS, emphasizing on-the-ground building of human resource capacity. The chapter concludes with observations drawn from a survey (commissioned by this committee) of American nongovernmental organizations engaged in HIV/AIDS projects in one or more PEPFAR focus countries (for a full report, see Appendix D).

THE PRESIDENT'S EMERGENCY PLAN
FOR AIDS RELIEF (PEPFAR)

As discussed in Chapter 1, PEPFAR, while encompassing activities in more than 100 countries, is focused on the development of comprehensive and integrated prevention, treatment, and care programs in 15 countries severely affected by HIV/AIDS. Box 3-1 presents the four cornerstones of the PEPFAR initiative. Key elements of the PEPFAR initiative include a Global AIDS Coordinator charged with supporting each national program using a country-specific approach, as well as coordinating U.S. and international actors (for example, bilateral donors, UN agencies, the Joint United Nations Programme on HIV/AIDS [UNAIDS], the Global Fund, and NGOs). Within the United States, the agencies primarily responsible for implementing PEPFAR are the U.S. Department of State (where the U.S. Global AIDS Coordinator is based and reports directly to the secretary of state); the

---

BOX 3-1
The Four Cornerstones of PEPFAR

1. Rapidly expanding *integrated prevention, treatment, and care* in the focus countries by using existing successful programs and building new ones that are needed.

2. Identifying *new partners,* including the private sector and faith- and community-based organizations, and building indigenous capacity to sustain a long-term and broad local response.

3. Encouraging *bold national leadership* in every impacted country around the world, and engendering the creation of sound, enabling policy environments in every country for combating HIV/AIDS and mitigating its consequences.

4. Implementing *strong strategic information systems* that will provide vital feedback and accountability, and help those fighting the epidemic in the PEPFAR countries to engage in continued learning and the identification of best practices.

United States Agency for International Development (USAID); and the U.S. Department of Health and Human Services (DHHS). Within DHHS, PEPFAR also draws on expertise from the National Institutes of Health/the National Institute for Allergy and Infectious Diseases (NIH/NIAID), which is involved in HIV/AIDS research in the PEPFAR focus countries; the Health Resources and Services Administration, which has experience expanding HIV/AIDS and other health services in resource-poor settings in the United States and is providing some assistance in several of the PEPFAR focus countries; and the Office of the Secretary/Office of Global Affairs, which plays a coordinating role for HIV/AIDS efforts within DHHS. Other agencies involved in PEPFAR include the Department of Defense, the Peace Corps, and the Departments of Labor and Commerce.

Recent Activities

PEPFAR is currently overseen by Ambassador Randall Tobias, the Global AIDS Coordinator, who was nominated by President Bush in July 2003 and confirmed by the Senate in October 2003. In February 2004, the Office of the Global AIDS Coordinator submitted a 5-year strategic plan to Congress and awarded its first $350 million in initial funding, including new awards to NGOs with established HIV/AIDS experience in the PEPFAR focus countries. In late 2004, U.S. embassies in the focus countries submitted detailed country operations plans both for fiscal year 2005 and for the 5-year period through fiscal year 2008. At the World Economic Forum held in Davos, Switzerland, in January 2005, it was announced that 172,000 individuals had received antiretroviral drugs under PEPFAR during its first 8 months, well within the range of the projected goal of 200,000 treated individuals over the first year of the initiative (O'Neill, 2005). In fiscal year 2004, the United States committed a total of $2.4 billion to the fight against global HIV/AIDS, and the projected amount for fiscal year 2005 is $2.8 billion. The budget request for fiscal year 2006 is $3.2 billion (O'Neill, 2005).

Widely acknowledged as the primary obstacle to achieving PEPFAR's 5-year goals in the hardest-hit nations (see Chapter 1) is their desperate lack of infrastructure and human resources. For this reason, a substantial portion of the U.S. funding is being invested in training health care workers, and in upgrading national and local public health infrastructure under national strategies.

Cooperation with other international donors is another key element of PEPFAR. In April 2004, in response to widespread concern that proliferating external funding streams were placing untenable demands on target country capacities, more than 20 donors, including the United States, Britain, and UNAIDS, announced their commitment to three principles for concerted action on HIV/AIDS, defined as "the three ones": one national HIV/AIDS authority including multisectoral and nongovernmental partners, one national strategy framework coordinating the work of all partners, and one monitoring and evaluation system in each country. Implementation of this agreement is intended to ensure that donors will work together while also recognizing that host nations must own the fight against HIV/AIDS.

Early Assessments

PEPFAR's strengths—its extraordinary leadership and financial commitment, swiftness, and focused efforts within a relatively small number of countries—have catalyzed hope and mobilized action within the current focus countries and partner agencies. Nonetheless, the challenges facing PEPFAR are great. Although positive overall, a May 2004 report by the Council on Foreign Relations (CFR) and the Milbank Memorial Fund (CFR and Milbank Memorial Fund, 2004) underscores three key issues:

- PEPFAR's underemphasis on infrastructure and human capital:

   The absence of hospitals, health centers, clinics, delivery services and other physical infrastructure has been crippling and will constitute a major obstacle to progress. The deficit in human capital—the health care workers necessary to treat, counsel, and care for patients, and to manage and administer health systems—has been debilitating and will continue to worsen. Many sub-Saharan countries . . . devote only a few dollars per capita per year to health; Ethiopia, for example, currently spends approximately $1. (p. 10)

- PEPFAR's underemphasis on testing:

> Whereas the five-year U.S. goal aims to get 2 million people on treatments, there are currently 20 million infected people in the 14 countries selected by PEPFAR. . . . Ninety-five percent of Africans and 95 percent of people infected globally do not know their HIV status. . . . Part of the reason for the lack of testing is the stigma attached to going to HIV/AIDS-specific centers for this purpose. Vast increases in health facilities, clinics and health care workers will be needed to provide the setting to test, treat, counsel, and care for all who need to be reached. (p. 11)

- PEPFAR's overemphasis on services designed to deliver antiretrovirals, draining resources from other areas of the health system and creating a parallel structure.

The CFR/Milbank report stresses the need for the Office of the Global AIDS Coordinator to maximize the integration of PEPFAR's infrastructure-related investments with overall national health systems, specifically addressing the tuberculosis (TB)/HIV copandemic more broadly, and incorporating malaria into the strategy:

> This would mean training health workers to deal with a broad range of health problems: developing delivery systems that can accommodate drugs other than [antiretrovirals]; enhancing the testing, treatment and counseling capacities of existing health centers and clinics as much as possible before establishing separate ones for HIV/AIDS; providing incentives to retain health professionals who are leaving for developed countries; and helping national governments to develop comprehensive health systems, rather than drawing resources purely for HIV/AIDS work. (p. 13)

Another early review of PEPFAR, conducted by the Center for Strategic and International Studies in collaboration with the Kaiser Family Foundation, raised concerns related to PEPFAR's large disbursement through a collection of disparate funding mechanisms not prepared to provide urgent responses; the need for real-time monitoring and evaluation, as well as longer-term progress reports based on reliable data systems; and the need to coordinate with non-HIV/AIDS disease control activities already in place in the PEPFAR focus countries, organized by other local and international groups (Nieburg et al., 2004). An additional concern, raised by Manyeke Sengwana of KwaZulu Natal University's Health Economics and HIV/AIDS Research Division (HEARD), is the potentially negative impact PEPFAR could have on other health programs, agency programs, and countries other than those on which PEPFAR is focused (Sengwana, 2004).

THE WORLD HEALTH ORGANIZATION'S 3 × 5 INITIATIVE[1]

On December 1, 2003, J.W. Lee, the new Director General of WHO, introduced a "detailed and concrete plan" for treating 3 million AIDS-infected patients by 2005. This plan, known as the 3 × 5 initiative emphasizes revised, simplified, and standardized guidelines for ART in resource-poor settings; support for buying, financing, and supplying antiretrovirals and diagnostic technology; and training strategies for health professionals and lay health workers.

According to the most recent progress report on the 3 × 5 intiative, released in December 2004 by the second half of 2004, the number of people on ART in developing and transitional countries had increased from 440,000 to an estimated 700,000 (WHO, 2004). This latter figure equals roughly 12 percent of the estimated 5.8 million people currently in need of treatment in developing and transitional countries (see Table 3-1). The 700,000 figure includes people receiving ART supported by the Global Fund, PEPFAR, the World Bank, and other partners.

Achieving the target of treating 3 million people by the end of 2005 will require that at least another 2.3 million people initiate treatment in 2005. In 2005, a total of 5.1 million adults who need treatment still are not receiving it; of these, 72 percent live in sub-Saharan Africa and 22 percent in Asia.

The 3 × 5 initiative has been critiqued from several perspectives: operational applications (including treatment guidelines, drug selection, manufacturing sources, rate of patient treatment, rate of drug resistance, regimen failure, drug procurements, human resources, and inconsistent figures on HIV/AIDS prevalence); price and cost implications; and ethical and legal consistency within the framework of the initiative. The initiative's overall intention is complicated by the fact that once AIDS treatment is initiated, those who finance and provide care become involved in chronic care management for the remainder of the patient's life.

On the other hand, one of the most innovative aspects of WHO's 3 × 5 initiative is a method for urgently training community health workers to support the delivery and monitoring of HIV/AIDS treatment (Jong-wook, 2003). An intensive training program can enable these health workers to evaluate and monitor patients and ensure that they receive and are taking their medicines. An example that involves training lay advocates or advisors to be community health workers is described in Box 3-2.

---

[1]This section draws heavily on WHO (2004).

TABLE 3-1 Estimated Number of People Receiving and Needing ART, and Percent Coverage in Developing and Transitional Countries by Region, December 2004

Region	Estimated Number of People Receiving ART, December 2004 (low estimate/high estimate)[a]	Estimated Number of People Aged 15–49 Needing ART[b]	ART Coverage (percent)[c]	Estimated Number of People Receiving ART
Sub-Saharan Africa	310,000 (270,000–350,000)	4,000,000	8	150,000
Latin America and the Caribbean	275,000 (260,000–290,000)	425,000	65	220,000
East, South, and Southeast Asia	100,000 (85,000–115,000)	1,200,000	8	55,000
Europe and Central Asia	15,000 (13,000–17,000)	150,000	10	11,000
North Africa and the Middle East[d]	4,000 (2,000–6,000)	55,000	7	4,000
Total	700,000 (630,000–780,000)	5,800,000	12	440,000

[a]A few countries report the number of children younger than age 15 receiving ART, and these children are included in this table. Preliminary data show that overall, these children represent less than 5 percent of the total number receiving ART.
[b]The figure presented is the midpoint of the low and high estimates of the number of AIDS deaths and the number of AIDS cases. Estimates for individual countries may differ according to the local methods used.
[c]This is a best coverage estimate based on the midpoints of the estimated numbers of people receiving and needing ART.
[d]Except for Turkey, no updates have been received from this region since June 2004.
NOTE: All countries except those in western Europe and Australia, Bahamas, Bahrain, Brunei, Canada, Cyrprus, Grenada, Israel, Japan, Kuwait, New Zealand, Qatar, Republic of Korea, Singapore, United Arab Emirates, and United States of America.
NOTE: Numbers do not add up due to rounding.
SOURCE: World Health Organization 3 by 5 Progress Report (2004:11).

BOX 3-2
**Community Health Workers: Augmenting Care for HIV/AIDS
and Tuberculosis in Haiti**

Community health workers are lay advocates or advisors who educate and lead individuals and groups in their communities to attain increased health and well-being. They act as bridges between the community and the providers of clinical health care services. Community health workers increase access to care by providing outreach and cultural linkages between their communities and clinical health care providers. They reduce the costs of health care by providing education, disease screening, and detection services that promote health and prevent disease. They often improve the health status of the community by providing primary health care at a low cost in remote areas.

Since 1987, Partners In Health and its sister organization Zanmi Lasante, Creole for "Partners In Health," have been providing primary health care in the central Haitian village of Cange. Together, they run a number of programs, including a full-service hospital, rural Haiti's only HIV/AIDS and tuberculosis treatment facilities, a women's health center, a dozen schools, and several cottage industries. In the Central Department of Haiti, where the partners work, there are fewer than two doctors per 100,000 persons. The population relies on community health workers to deliver care. Partners In Health and Zanmi Lasante trained 750 community health workers in 2003 alone. After training, these community health workers can provide basic medical diagnoses, treatment, and if necessary, referrals to clinics. They can also provide a variety of home-based support services, including directly observed therapy for HIV/AIDS and tuberculosis. It has been noted that adherence rates of these patients are high. Based on these successful experiences, community health workers appear to be an excellent option for the future of health care in resource-poor settings, especially for the management of diseases such as HIV/AIDS.

SOURCE: http://www.pih.org/wherewework/haiti/index.html and PIH annual report.

THE UNITED NATIONS GLOBAL FUND

In 2001, Kofi Annan, secretary general of the United Nations, proposed the Global Fund, a public–private partnership that would raise and disburse millions of dollars every year, to fight AIDS, TB, and malaria. The Global Fund aspires to be the world's largest fundraising and grant-making operation. Its governance and working methods were developed during the last few months of 2001, and its first grants were announced at the end of April 2002.

Among the guiding principles of the Global Fund is the notion of national ownership. In practice, applications for funding need to be endorsed by a group of people, known collectively as the Country Coordinating Mechanism (CCM), which typically includes a government representative. Such partnerships help facilitate local coordination, but they can also hinder access to funding by subgroups of HIV-infected stakeholders already marginalized within their own country, or by groups proposing public health interventions incongruent with government policies (Kerr et al., 2004).

By December 2004, the Global Fund had received pledges for U.S. $5.9 billion and payments of U.S. $3.3 billion against those pledges (WHO, 2004). In four rounds of disbursements, it has already approved proposals with a 2-year value of U.S. $3.1 billion and disbursed U.S. $860 million. Of the U.S. $3.1 billion approved, U.S. $1.7 billion (56 percent) has been allocated to the fight against AIDS with 70 percent going to low-income countries and 58 percent to sub-Saharan Africa.

More than half of the Global Fund's grants to date have been allocated to national governments; 25 percent to nongovernmental and community-based organizations; 4 percent to associations of people living with HIV/AIDS; and 5 percent each to academic institutions, the private sector, faith-based organizations, and others.

EFFORTS OF OTHER ORGANIZATIONS

The World Bank

Since 1995, The World Bank has committed more than U.S. $1.7 billion through grants, loans, and credits to support programs to combat HIV/AIDS (World Bank, 2005). More than U.S. $1 billion has gone to support the Multi-Country HIV/AIDS Program for Africa for 28 high-burden countries in that region and another U.S. $155 million has gone to the Caribbean Multi-Country HIV/AIDS Prevention and Control Adaptable Program Lending. The goal of these programs is to intensify action against HIV/AIDS in as many countries as possible and on all fronts, including prevention, testing, counseling, treatment, care, and support.

Between July and December 2004, the World Bank supported accelerated access to treatment through ongoing financial and technical support for improving national health systems in 100 countries. It also provided direct support to ART programs in the Caribbean, 13 African countries, 3 Asian countries, and 1 country in Eastern Europe.

In mid-2004, the World Bank announced the Treatment Acceleration Project; a U.S. $60 million International Development Association grant was provided to support scaling up of access to HIV/AIDS treatment in Burkina Faso, Ghana, and Mozambique. Another U.S. $15 million grant was given to Mali. Grassroots organizations, private companies such as the Private Enterprise Foundation/Pharma Access International in Ghana, faith-based groups such as the Community of Sant' Egidio in Mozambique, and a network of people living with HIV/AIDS in Burkina Faso are also involved in implementing the project, building on progress previously achieved on a smaller scale in partnership with ministries of health.

THE UNITED STATES AGENCY FOR INTERNATIONAL DEVELOPMENT

In fiscal year 2003, the budget of the USAID for global HIV/AIDS programs was $795 million, allocated to more than 50 of the most affected developing countries worldwide (USAID, 2005a). Since the announcement of PEPFAR, USAID's work in fighting HIV/AIDS has come under a new mandate. The agency's global HIV/AIDS grants are currently available through the following programs:

• **Communities Responding to the HIV/AIDS Epidemic (CORE) Initiative**—Through CORE, USAID provides small grants to community and faith-based groups in developing countries. Priority is given to groups that commit their own resources, and that demonstrate the ability to meet needs for care and support (especially care for orphans and vulnerable children) and to help confront and reduce stigma and discrimination (Core Initiative, 2005).
• **Community Rapid and Effective Action Combating HIV/AIDS (REACH)**—Community REACH provides grants, typically ranging from $100,000 to $500,000 over 1 to 3 years, to organizations such as regional and local NGOs, universities, and faith-based organizations involved in primary prevention and education, voluntary counseling and testing, and care for those living with HIV/AIDS (Pact, 2005).
• **Child Survival and Health Grants Programs**—This funding mechanism, open to any U.S.-based private voluntary organization, supports community-oriented child survival programs. These programs can involve initiatives targeting HIV/AIDS and support for orphans and vulnerable children (USAID, 2005b).

The U.S. Department of Health and Human Services/Health Resources and Services Administration

Through an intradepartmental delegation of authority from the Centers for Disease Control and Prevention (CDC), HRSA is currently charged with increasing access to international HIV/AIDS treatment, care, and support (HRSA, 2005). Examples of activities focused on fostering human resources for health include the International AIDS Education and Training Center on HIV (I-TECH; see below), an HRSA-supported program designed to achieve rapid expansion of the pool of trained providers, managers, and allied health staff providing HIV/AIDS, malaria, and tuberculosis (TB) services in developing countries; and the American International Health Alliance (AIHA; see below), the lead organization currently overseeing the HRSA-supported HIV/AIDS Twinning Center and launching the Voluntary Healthcare Corps under PEPFAR.

International Training and Education Center on HIV

I-TECH, a collaboration of the University of Washington and the University of California, San Francisco, was initially funded by HRSA and CDC's Control and Prevention Global AIDS Program (GAP) in 2002, and since 2003 has additionally been funded by USAID for work in the Caribbean. Its mission is to promote activities that increase human capacity for HIV/AIDS clinical care and support in countries and regions hardest hit by the HIV/AIDS pandemic (Holmes, 2004; I-TECH, 2005). I-TECH is currently working with GAP and local partners in Botswana, Ethiopia, Haiti, India, Namibia, Malawi, South Africa, Thailand, and Zimbabwe and has launched start-up activities in Guyana and Vietnam. Its principal focus is training, encompassing the following:

- Level I: Didactic activities (grand rounds, clinic conferences, day-long lecture series)
- Level II: Skill building (role plays, case studies)
- Level III: Hands-on clinical training (mentorship, mini-residencies)
- Level IV: Clinical consultation (phone, videoconference, e-mail, mobile team visits)

I-TECH emphasizes training models for both physicians and nurses, recognizing that the latter provide the majority of HIV/AIDS care overseas and require both technical knowledge and empowerment.

American International Health Alliance

AIHA defines twinning as "a voluntary, formal, sustainable partnership between two or more similar organizations established to collaborate in providing technical assistance on HIV prevention, care, and treatment through exchange visits, training, and ongoing communications and organization support" (AIHA, 2005). AIHA-managed twinning partnerships will typically link U.S. and PEPFAR focus country partners, although partnerships between focus countries (south–south) with or without a third country (trilateral) can also be supported. With technical assistance on HIV/AIDS treatment and care provided by I-TECH, anticipated activities of AIHA twinning partnerships include needs assessments; baseline data sur-

veys; professional exchanges, training, and mentoring; development of curricula and other educational/training material; and scaling up or replication
of successful treatment, care, and support programs. Organizations that
may engage in twinning include community- and faith-based programs and
clinics; hospitals or health posts; public health programs; schools of medicine, nursing, allied health, pharmacy, public health, management, public
administration, etc.; HIV/AIDS education and training programs; AIDS
service organizations; and others, depending on host country needs (Smith,
2005).

A second program area of AIHA is the Voluntary Healthcare Corps
(VHC), currently conceived as a network of individuals with expertise in
health care and HIV/AIDS who will work in established twinning partnerships or in programs in other PEPFAR focus countries. Assignments will
range from 3 months to 3 years, although most are expected to last 3 to 6
months (Smith, 2005).

The Centers for Disease Control and Prevention

CDC works collaboratively to mitigate global HIV/AIDS with other
U.S. government agencies, including USAID; international health and economic organizations such as WHO, UNAIDS, and the World Bank; NGOs;
and host country governments. From having had no HIV/AIDS funding in
1999, CDC currently has a $500 million portfolio of projects focused on
global HIV/AIDS. In 2004, these projects were staffed by 103 direct hires
(Civil Service/Commissioned Corps) in Atlanta and 100 in the field (coun-
try/regional programs), as well as contractors, fellows, and other skilled
personnel in Atlanta and overseas (St. Louis, 2004). In 2003, GAP operated
in 25 countries in Africa, Asia, Latin America, and the Caribbean, with
regional offices/activities located in the Caribbean, Southeast Asia, Southern Africa, and Central America. GAP has three primary program foci:
infrastructure and capacity development, including surveillance, laboratory
support, information systems, and monitoring and evaluation; primary prevention, including voluntary counseling and testing, blood safety, and
youth-targeted activities; and care and treatment, including treatment and
care of TB and opportunistic infections, prevention of mother-to-child transmission, appropriate provision of antiretroviral drugs, and soothing care
(CDC, 2005).

Many of CDC's cooperative agreements support expatriate human
resources for health; these include the University Technical Assistance Program, I-TECH, the Association of Public Health Laboratories, and the
National Association of State and Territorial AIDS Directors. A new model
for international deployments is the Global AIDS fellowship (cosponsored
by the American Schools of Public Health). The program attracted 63 ap-

plicants for 10 postings in 2005, most of whom had international experience plus a recent masters degree in public health (St. Louis, 2004).

Research Programs Supported by the National Institutes of Health

Early clinical and translational research investments by NIH contributed to the development of university- and community-based centers of excellence throughout the United States around which most of the initial comprehensive AIDS care centers developed. These centers (primarily the Adult and Pediatric AIDS Clinical Trials Group, the Community Program for Clinical Research on AIDS, the HIV Prevention Trials Network, the HIV Vaccine Trials Network, and the Centers for AIDS Research) enabled the development of comprehensive care programs that ultimately yielded the knowledge base that has drastically changed the prognosis of the disease.

Similar NIH-funded programs are now operating in a variety of resource-limited settings, including PEPFAR focus countries. These programs have invested in the training of local investigators and clinicians through structured twinning between American academic centers and international sites; they have also provided equipment (such as flow cytometers and polymerase chain reaction [PCR] equipment) serving dual goals of research and care. In addition to providing infrastructure and training, such programs enable local investigators to frame research questions and conduct research designed to optimize local care. The research addresses, for example, approaches to preventing mother-to-child transmission of HIV that do not compromise the subsequent responsiveness of the mother to therapy, optimizing ART in treatment-naïve and -experienced patients, and monitoring and managing drug resistance.[2]

NIH's Fogarty International Center (FIC) recently launched the International Clinical, Operational, and Health Services Research Training Award for AIDS and Tuberculosis (ICOHRTA-AIDS/TB). The program is designed to provide extended support to training institutions in low- and middle-income country sites where HIV/AIDS and TB or both are significant problems (Fogarty International Center, 2004). ICOHRTA-AIDS/TB is intended to build capacity for integrated clinical, operational, and health

---

[2]Examples of such studies include AIDS Clinical Trial Group (ACTG) study 5175, which will test novel once-daily antiretroviral drug regimens in 1,200 individuals living in resource-limited settings; ACTG 5207, which seeks to delineate approaches for reducing drug resistance in mothers receiving single-dose nevirapine to prevent mother-to-child HIV transmission; and ACTG 5208, which addresses the extent to which prior perinatal nevirapine compromises a mother's response to subsequent ART (R. Schooley, personal communication, February 14, 2005).

services research across the full range of conditions and issues that relate to care of adult and pediatric patients with HIV/AIDS or TB by a wide range of health professionals (e.g., nurses, midwives, physicians, dentists, health care administrators, and public health workers).

With eight NIH partners, FIC also operates the Global Health Research Initiative Program for New Foreign Investigators. This program promotes the reentry of young NIH-trained foreign investigators from the developing world to their home countries, thus ensuring that developing countries do not lose their talented scientists.

Foundations and Corporate Initiatives[3]

The Bill and Melinda Gates Foundation has focused considerable attention on HIV/AIDS since its founding in January 2000, allocating $250 million annually. The emphasis on HIV vaccine research and new technologies, such as female microbicides, that could block the sexual transmission of HIV. The Gates Foundation is the only private-sector organization to make a significant cash donation ($100 million) to the Global Fund.

Beginning in 2003, President Clinton, through the William Jefferson Clinton Foundation and numerous volunteer experts, contracted with selected African and Latin American countries (and, most recently, China) to broker low-cost, high-volume delivery of generic drugs and diagnostic equipment. The Clinton Foundation also provides short- and medium-term expert teams to assist countries in preparing detailed operations plans for scaling up national treatment programs.

Corporate employers such as DaimlerChrysler, Anglo American, DeBeers, Standard Charter Bank, Coca Cola, Merck, and India's Tata and Iron and Steel with a significant presence in the southern African epicenter of the pandemic have spearheaded innovative programs in response to rising rates of HIV infection among their own workers. Drug companies such as Merck, GlaxoSmithKline, and Bristol-Myers Squibb have established reduced-price, no-profit, or free drug programs in many highly affected countries.

The Pfizer Global Health Fellows program is an innovative response that goes beyond conventional industry donations of cash and drugs (see Box 3-3). First announced at the International AIDS Conference in Barcelona in 2002, it provides a mechanism for sending Pfizer employees with relevant medical and managerial expertise to support the work of leading NGOs such as Doctors of the World, the Elizabeth Glazer Pediatric AIDS Foundation, the American Jewish World Service, the African Medi-

---

[3]Much of the information in this section is drawn from Morrison (2004).

BOX 3-3
Pfizer Fellows

Since 2002, 51 Fellows have been deployed from 15 Pfizer sites to 18 countries. The company's newest Global Health Fellows program sends skilled Pfizer
medical and managerial volunteers to help nongovernmental organizations
(NGOs) develop the health and social infrastructures required to combat HIV/AIDS
in developing countries. To this end, Pfizer loans skilled employees to NGOs for up
to 6 months while paying the employees' salaries and keeping their jobs open until
they return. Pfizer also covers the cost of assignment, including NGO overhead;
provides orientation and cultural sensitivity training to Fellows; manages the application process and initial screening of applicants; provides logistical support to
Fellows prior to their deployment; and demonstrates the value of the program to
Fellows' Pfizer managers.

The partnering NGOs are responsible for identifying field needs. They then
develop job descriptions and select the fellows they wish to work with from a pool
of applicants. The NGOs also manage the Fellows in the field, including identifying
housing, transportation, and logistics related to the Fellows' assignments. At the
end of an assignment, the NGO assesses the Fellow's performance as part of the
partnership evaluation process.

SOURCE: Pfizer (2003).

---

cal and Research Foundation, the Academic Alliance for AIDS Care and
Prevention in Africa, and Health Volunteers Overseas (Pfizer, 2003). The
company sees its effort as a way to apply global pharmaceutical corporate
know-how to the greater needs of society through a cross-sector collaboration.

Pfizer also donates medicines through its Diflucan[4] Partnership Program and partnered with the Academic Alliance for AIDS Care and Prevention in Africa to build a new Infectious Diseases Institute (IDI) on the
campus of Makerere University in Kampala, Uganda. Completed in 2004,
the new facility is already serving as a training center for hundreds of
physicians working on HIV/AIDS care and prevention in Africa. Currently,
two infectious disease specialists vetted by the Infectious Diseases Society of
America go to IDI every 9 weeks and teach back-to-back 1-month courses
for physicians. Applicants are selected on the basis of their potential to train
others after completing the program. IDI also provides 1-week and week-
end training programs for nurses and other health professionals and main-

---

[4]Diflucan™, or fluconazole, is an antifungal drug used to treat cryptococcosis, an opportunistic fungal infection that frequently causes meningitis in AIDS patients.

tains on ground-the-clock AIDS Treatment Information Center staffed by pharmacists and physicians who respond to questions by phone, fax, and e-mail (Scheld, 2004).

Other U.S. Private-Sector, Academic, and Faith- and Community-Based Programs

In addition to the initiatives described above, many innovative programs focused on global HIV/AIDS have been initiated by other U.S. private-sector, academic, and faith- and community-based organizations. Certain programs that emphasize training and augmentation of human health care resources are described in greater detail in Chapter 5.

The committee commissioned an independent survey of lessons learned from a range of nongovernmental sending organizations involved in HIV/AIDS activities in at least one PEPFAR focus country. During the committee's February 2005 meeting, the findings of this survey were reported. The survey encompassed U.S. faith-based or secular NGOs with budgets of between $100,000 and $1.5 billion. In general, the larger organizations surveyed perceive HIV/AIDS as a "low to medium" issue as compared with relief for the recent tsunami in the Indian Ocean. This view reflects the projected duration of involvement on the ground for the two efforts (3–4 years following the tsunami versus 30 years or more for HIV/AIDS). Most of the surveyed organizations send volunteer doctors and nurses (as opposed to administrators, human resources personnel, information technologists, laboratory workers, or public health specialists) for less than 2 months. In some cases, however, there is a U.S. "anchor-person" who can inform future volunteers, as well as maintain ongoing electronic contact with overseas colleagues and counterparts.

Additional ground-level challenges cited by the surveyed organizations were as follows:

- Partnering challenges
  — Local operating obstacles (e.g., obtaining a permit to operate a truck)
  — Lack of clarity regarding project goals
  — Lack of local supervision of volunteers
  — Dependency on local partners[5]
  — Negative local reactions to the size, perceived dominance, arrogance, and/or resources of very large organizations

---

[5]For example, in some cases American health professionals may attract more patients than indigenous providers because they are perceived to have superior knowledge and skills.

- Issues pertaining to local skills and infrastructure
  — Unexpected expenses
  — Lack of local strategic planning skills
  — Lack of local project evaluation skills
  — Inadequate work space
  — High turnover of indigenous staff

- Contextual issues
  — Chronic community depression over HIV/AIDS and other survival challenges, including local civil conflicts
  — Potential for personal isolation of volunteers
  — Impact of desperate overall situation on volunteers

- Issues pertaining to international bureaucracy: overevaluation of projects

REFERENCES

AIHA (American International Health Alliance). 2005. *HIV/AIDS Twinning Center Frequently Asked Questions.* [Online]. Available: http://www.twinningagainstaids.org/faq.html [accessed March 1, 2005].

Anabwani G, Navario P. 2005. Nutrition and HIV/AIDS in sub-Saharan Africa: An overview. *Nutrition* 21(1):96–99.

CDC (Centers for Disease Control and Prevention). 2005. *Global AIDS Program.* [Online]. Available: http://www.cdc.gov/nchstp/od/gap/default.htm [accessed March 1, 2005].

CFR (Council on Foreign Relations) and Milbank Memorial Fund. 2004. *Addressing the HIV/AIDS Pandemic: A U.S. Global AIDS Strategy for the Long Term.* New York, NY: Milbank Memorial Fund.

Core Initiative. 2005. *Communities Responding to the HIV/AIDS Epidemic.* [Online]. Available: http://www.coreinitiative.org [accessed March 1, 2005].

Fogarty International Center. 2004. *FAQ: International Clinical, Operational, and Health Services Research Training Award Program for AIDS and Tuberculosis.* [Online]. Available: http://www.fic.nih.gov/news/FAQ113004.html [accessed March 1, 2005].

Holmes K. 2004 (December 1). *Model of Training for Grassroots Work in HIV.* Presentation at the December 1, 2004, Workshop of the IOM Committee on the Overseas Placement of U.S. Health Professionals, Washington, DC.

HRSA (Health Resources and Services Administration). 2005. *Global HIV/AIDS Program.* [Online]. Available: http://hab.hrsa.gov/special/global.htm [accessed March 1, 2005].

I-TECH (International Training and Education Center on HIV). 2005. *I-TECH.* [Online]. Available: http://www.go2itech.org/itech?page=home-00-00 [accessed March 1, 2005].

IRINnews. 2004. *Southern Africa: Are Countries Spending Enough on HIV/AIDS?* [Online]. Available: http://www.irinnews.org/report.asp?ReportID=38932&SelectRegion=SouthernAfrica &SelectCountry=SOUTHERN_AFRICA [accessed March 1, 2005].

Jong-wook L. 2003. Global health improvement and WHO: Shaping the future. *Lancet* 362:2083–2088.

Kerr T, Kaplan K, Suwannawong P, Jurgens R, Wood E. 2004. The Global Fund to fight AIDS, tuberculosis and malaria: Funding for unpopular public-health programmes. *Lancet* 364:11–12.

Morrison JS. 2004. *HIV/AIDS Pandemic and U.S. Leadership.* [Online]. Available: http://www.aspeninstitute.org/admin/index.asp?downloadid=1229 [accessed March 1, 2005].

Nieburg P, Kates J, Morrison JS. 2004. *Enhancing the Rapid Response Capacity of the U.S. Global AIDS Coordinator: Lessons Learned from Other U.S. Emergency Responses.* Washington, DC: Center for Strategic and International Studies.

O'Neill J. 2005 (February 14). *The Charge to the Committee.* Presentation at the February 14, 2005, Workshop of the IOM Committee on Options for the Overseas Placement of U.S. Health Professionals, Washington, DC.

Pact. 2005. *Community REACH.* [Online]. Available: http://www.pactworld.org/reach [accessed March 1, 2005].

Pfizer. 2003. *Pfizer Global Health Fellows Program Sends Company Volunteers to Work with NGOs to Fight HIV/AIDS in Developing Countries.* [Online]. Available: http://www.pfizer.com/subsites/philanthropy/news/mn_2003_0612.html [accessed March 1, 2005].

Scheld WM. 2004 (December 2). *Academic Alliance for AIDS Care and Prevention in Africa.* Presentation at the December 2, 2004, Workshop of the IOM Committee on Options for the Overseas Placement of U.S. Health Professionals, Washington, DC.

Sengwana M. 2004. *Review of 'the President's Emergency Plan for AIDS Relief.'* Durban, South Africa: University of KwaZulu-Natal. [Online]. Available: http://www.ukzn.ac.za/heard/research/ResearchReports/2004/PEPFAR percent20BRIEFING percent20NOTE percent20Final percent2021 percent20Sept04.pdf [accessed March 18, 2005].

Smith J. 2005 (February 14). *Working in a PEPFAR Context.* Presentation at the February 14, 2005, Workshop of the IOM Committee on Options for the Overseas Placement of U.S. Health Professionals, Washington, DC.

St. Louis M. 2004 (December 2). *USPHS-CDC.* Presentation at the December 2, 2004, Workshop of the IOM Committee on Options for the Overseas Placement of U.S. Health Professionals, Washington, DC.

UNAIDS (Joint United Nations Programme on HIV/AIDS). 2003. *International Funding for HIV/AIDS.* [Online]. Available: http://www.unaids.org.ungass/en/global/UNGASS05_en.html [accessed March 1, 2005].

USAID (U.S. Agency for International Development). 2005a. *HIV/AIDS Funding: Frequently Asked Questions.* [Online]. Available: http://www.usaid.gov/our_work/global_health/aids/Funding/fundingfaq.html [accessed March 1, 2005].

USAID. 2005b. *Child Survival & Health Grants Program.* [Online]. Available: http://www.usaid.gov/our_work/global_health/home/Funding/cs_grants/cs_index.html [accessed March 1, 2005].

WHO (World Health Organization). 2004. *3 by 5 Progress Report.* Geneva, Switzerland: WHO. [Online]. Available: http://www.who.int/3by5/en/ProgressReportfinal.pdf [accessed March 4, 2005].

World Bank. 2005. *Intensifying Action Against AIDS in Africa.* [Online]. Available: http://www.worldbank.org/afr/aids/ [accessed March 4, 2005].

4

Envisioning a U.S. Global Health Service

This chapter presents the organizing framework for a new suite of programs and activities designed to respond to the PEPFAR mandate, and to contribute knowledge and expertise on the ground to fight HIV/AIDS, as well as tuberculosis (TB), malaria, and other global scourges. In proposing this group of programs, the committee aims to help address the grave deficiency of human health care resources in countries targeted by PEPFAR, leveraging and multiplying local responses on the ground. The committee's proposals reflect a recognition of the pivotal contributions that U.S. health workers can make in partnership with overseas colleagues in the common fight against these terrible diseases.

As the overall implementing mechanism for these proposals, the committee envisions a Global Health Service (GHS), as detailed in this chapter. The six specific programs proposed for the GHS—a corps of experts, needs assessment, a competitive 1-year fellowship program, a loan repayment program, organizational twinning, and a clearinghouse—are discussed in Chapter 5.

Recommendation 1: *Create a U.S. Global Health Service.* The committee discussed the importance of establishing a clear identity for programs designed to mobilize health personnel for service in combating HIV/AIDS in highly impacted countries. A well recognized identity—a brand—was felt to be essential to the creation of mission and the promotion of volunteerism. **Therefore the committee recommends the establishment of a U.S. Global Health Service to serve as the umbrella organization for the initiatives and programs to be proposed in this report.**

Recommendation 1a: *Mobilize providers and capacity developers.* The committee believes that a wide variety of health professionals and other key technical and management personnel will be essential for achieving the PEPFAR goals of treating 2 million HIV-infected people, preventing 7 million new HIV infections, and caring for 10 million HIV-affected individuals and vulnerable children (the 2-7-10 PEPFAR goals), as well as for building the long-term capacity necessary to control HIV/AIDS, tuberculosis, and malaria. **Therefore, the committee recommends that the programs of the U.S. Global Health Service initially focus on the mobilization of clinicians, technicians, and management personnel in direct response to specified in-country needs to achieve PEPFAR goals. In view of the lack of human resources for health in PEPFAR focus countries and many other developing countries, education, training, and development of new, effective configurations of health care delivery in resource-poor settings will take high priority among the U.S. Global Health Service's activities.**

VISION AND MISSION

The desire to perform volunteer service was first noted as a distinctly American trait by Alexis de Tocqueville in the early nineteenth century. Multiple examples since that time attest to the service and compassion of many Americans toward fellow citizens at home and around the world. Today, an unprecedented medical tragedy offers a new opportunity for Americans to give and give back. The vision behind the committee's proposal for the GHS springs from a shared conviction that health is a human right, and one that can be attained in a global context only through the coordinated efforts of committed partners.

The mission of the GHS is to be flexible and responsive to the needs for human resources for health identified by countries whose citizens are most affected by the HIV/AIDS pandemic and other global scourges; to provide expertise in the form of caregivers, technical advisers, trainers, and mentors; and to sustain enduring relationships after working with colleagues on the ground.

Why "Global Health" and Not Just "HIV/AIDS"

The committee understood that the participants and programs it envisioned would have, as their primary agenda, a commitment to helping PEPFAR reach its ambitious 5-year goals (i.e., providing antiretroviral therapy [ART] for 2 million people; preventing 7 million new HIV infections; and providing care to 10 million people infected with or affected by

HIV/AIDS, including orphans and vulnerable children). The committee endorsed the PEPFAR goals and agreed that they should guide its recommendations. At the same time, considering the daily realities of health care in many settings in PEPFAR countries, the committee also concluded that some GHS participants would need to possess knowledge, skills, and experience extending beyond HIV/AIDS. For example, participants might partner with host country colleagues in the direct provision of clinical care and treatment or end-of-life palliative care for HIV/AIDS patients, provide pharmacy or laboratory support, perform training functions, help redesign infrastructure and health systems, or provide other forms of technical assistance within the public or private health sectors of targeted countries.

From a purely medical perspective, multiple overlapping diseases associated with poverty (especially TB and malaria; see Chapter 1) and other primary care needs coexist among HIV-infected and vulnerable populations in developing countries. As discussed in Chapter 2, entry points for HIV/AIDS care include, among others, voluntary counseling and testing sites, primary care clinics, sexual and reproductive health services, and hospitals. At more advanced stages of infection, the comprehensive care of HIV/AIDS patients requires not only mastery of ART and monitoring, but also diagnostic and management expertise pertaining to TB; skin, lung, intestinal, and bloodstream infections; sexually transmitted infections, and other opportunistic infections. In addition, parasitic diseases—most notably malaria—and nutritional issues threaten the health and survival of HIV/AIDS patients and vulnerable populations in developing countries.

In short, HIV/AIDS care cannot be isolated from the health context in developing countries, nor should there be parallel programs of HIV/AIDS-related and -nonrelated care in health systems already limited in capacity. In the worst-case scenario, the former could actually detract from the latter, leading to the unintended negative consequence of an even greater disease burden within the general population. For this reason, U.S. health providers sent to work in a particular developing country will need an understanding of its situation with regard to HIV/AIDS-related diseases, as well as HIV/AIDS itself.

Another factor influencing the committee's thinking was the setting in which U.S. health professionals would work in PEPFAR focus countries. GHS participants will need to understand and accept the challenges and frustrations of delivering health care in resource-poor settings, while at the same time maintaining positive, supportive attitudes toward colleagues and patients, a committed engagement in the tasks they perform, and an overall attitude of service. Simply put, the individuals participating in the GHS as envisioned by the committee will need not only expertise, but also personal attributes qualifying them as outstanding global ambassadors and coworkers on the ground.

Taking all of these factors into account, the committee concluded that the term "Global Health Service" most accurately conveys the master program's immediate portfolio of activity and expertise, as well as its long-term goal of helping to advance population health in target countries. Another consideration in choosing the name "Global Health Service" was the potential stigma associated with "HIV Corps," one alternative considered by the committee. Stigma has major negative impacts on health-seeking behavior, especially among patients at risk for HIV/AIDS. Despite the best intentions of its sponsors and participants, a new program with a stigmatizing name could potentially discourage individual patients or whole communities from fully embracing its mission or functions.

Linking "Global Health" and "Service"

Creating a culture of service was a primary motivation behind the committee's proposal for a new, federally funded initiative to help to address the human resource crisis in addressing global HIV/AIDS. The needs for service within global health arena are obvious. Despite remarkable advances in health over the last century, the poorest people in the world still suffer heavy burdens of misery and premature death. They should know that others in the world care about their plight. They also need tangible help in the form of global medical aid. Without human health care resources, however, aid—whether in the form of money, drugs, or investments in physical infrastructure—will not achieve its maximum desired impact.

Many U.S. health workers identify the desire to help others as a primary motivation in their original choice of profession and currently engage in service activities in their work and personal lives. However, some would like to make an even larger contribution by serving internationally. In a world of growing disparities between the healthy "haves" and "have-nots," the desires and talents of these Americans deserve a meaningful avenue for expression.

Moreover, the next generation of health care workers is increasingly interested in global health. More than 20 percent of students graduating from U.S. medical schools in 2003 participated in an international health experience during their undergraduate medical training, compared with just 6 percent of students graduating in 1984 (AAMC, 1984, 2003). The committee envisions that such individuals—in many health fields—will carry the mission of the GHS forward.

Finally, many health workers on the front lines of the battle against the HIV/AIDS pandemic and global diseases associated with poverty are already serving beyond the call of duty. Despite concerns about their own physical safety, economic security, and psychological stress, these individuals continue to display enormous dedication and fortitude in the pursuit of their mission. They need allies. Inspired by their service, the committee embraced the concept of global collaboration in service as the catalyst and central unifying principle for the GHS.

Unitary Management and Values

As envisioned by the committee, the GHS encompasses a suite of programs under a single banner. Multiple administrative arrangements could be envisioned for the GHS programs. A variety of organizations, whose attributes are listed in Appendix G, could be considered as models. However, the committee members were in agreement that the parent program should be housed within the U.S. government, although certain activities and functions might be contracted to experienced nongovernmental organizations (NGOs).

Strategic justifications for housing the individual programs proposed for the GHS within the federal government are presented in Chapter 5. In general, the committee believes that a government-based program will enhance the international credibility, transparency, and clarity of purpose of the GHS; position it closer to the federal appropriations process; and enable certain of its key functions. In addition, a single management structure will serve as a focal point for legislation, budgeting, and administration while allowing the parent office to maximize efficiency and streamline operations. Notwithstanding these conclusions on the importance of the governmental anchor of the GHS, the committee believes that the use of private-sector contracts and public–private partnering will be crucial to foster creative solutions, to supplement financing, and to enhance administrative flexibility.

> **Recommendation 2:** *Manage the programs of the U.S. Global Health Service in a unitary fashion.* The committee recommends that the programs of the U.S. Global Health Service be managed in a unitary fashion to provide maximum synergy, coordination, and clarity of purpose. Fiscal, administrative, and management matters should be handled by the single organizational entity that would be dedicated to the mission of mobilizing U.S. personnel to work in PEPFAR focus countries. Finally, in order for the U.S. Global Health Service to relate closely to PEPFAR and to participate in the annual federal budget process, the committee recommends that the U.S. Global Health Service should be a program of the federal government. In order to be successful, the U.S. Global Health Service needs to collaborate with the private sector, NGOs, and public–private matching programs.

Public input to the management of such a high-visibility global program is important for maintaining a balanced view. The committee believes that the best mechanism to this end would be an external advisory committee. Recognizing the fundamental importance of involving partners in the development and ongoing operation of the GHS, the committee believes further that the members of the advisory committee should include colleagues from the PEPFAR focus countries and NGOs, as well as other key collaborators from the United States and abroad.

Recommendation 2a: *Establish an advisory committee for the Global Health Service that includes international members.* The committee recognizes the fundamental importance of involving partners in the development and ongoing operation of the U.S. Global Health Service. These partners would include colleagues from nongovernmental organizations, PEPFAR countries, and other key collaborators from the United States and abroad. **The committee recommends the creation of a policy-level advisory committee with international colleagues and a commitment to the strategic engagement of public and private partners in the planning, operation, and evaluation of the U.S. Global Health Service.**

While a variety of programs to mobilize U.S. health professionals for service abroad are already in existence, none encompasses the scope and values of the proposed GHS, which include the following:

- A portfolio of human resource capacity-building mechanisms that individually provide unique benefits and together create synergistic benefits otherwise not possible
- Opportunities for strategic, multifaceted deployment relating to the operating plans of PEPFAR countries
- Possibilities for strategic public–private partnerships within and among countries that are both federally funded and benefit from funding and resources from other sectors
- National prominence for volunteering opportunities
- Reduction of barriers to developing governmental relationships among countries and collaboration among agencies within the United States
- Coordinated responsibility and accountability for target setting and performance monitoring

PRINCIPLES AND MERIT FRAMEWORK

The GHS as envisioned by the committee is framed by a set of six guiding principles. These principles are detailed below.

Country responsiveness. The programs and members of the GHS will at all times support and be responsive to the host countries in which they operate in both the public and private health sectors. Under the full-time/ long-term program proposed by the committee (the Global Health Service Corps, discussed in Chapter 5), countries will actually trigger deployments (according to the operations plans of PEPFAR countries and/or national internal needs assessments) from among a range of specialists and expertise. Thus the committee endorsed the concept of local ownership (see below), with the support provided being tailored to specific settings, and ongoing monitoring and evaluation being carried out for quality improvement.

Interdisciplinary, cross-cutting approach. The effective provision of HIV/AIDS prevention and treatment services, as well as other control efforts targeting major global diseases, requires the talents and expertise of many skilled professionals, including, for example, clinicians (doctors, nurses, and other care providers), public health specialists, laboratory personnel, pharmacists, information technologists, and health systems managers and planners. The committee stresses the need for interdisciplinary and cross-cutting approaches so that the GHS can respond flexibly and creatively to diverse needs on the ground.

Training for self-sufficiency. The long-term goal of the GHS is not to provide U.S. health professionals as permanent substitutes for local workers or even to augment local forces, but to empower receiving countries. A key factor in empowerment is training for self-sufficiency. In the long run, self-sufficiency in health care will develop incrementally, nurtured by many investments. With respect to human resources for health, however, the committee envisions self-sufficiency developing on a foundation of professional and institutional relationships. Following overseas service, cross-border personal networks will continue to foster self-sufficiency and collegial exchanges.

Nondepletion of the local health care workforce. The committee recognizes that depletion or diversion of the current health workforce in PEPFAR focus countries could inadvertently result from a well-intentioned global health program on the ground. The GHS will engage in ongoing monitoring of its impact on local health care to ensure that it does not drain resources from essential local services or foster the international migration of health workers.

Multiplier effect. To the extent possible, participants in programs of the GHS will pursue the goal of cost-effective force multiplication. Given the dire lack of human resources for health in many developing countries, investments in education, training, and new effective approaches to health care delivery will take priority among the activities of the Global Health Service Corps. Such efforts may be further augmented by long-distance learning programs and modern information and network technology, which could eventually encompass a collection of physically dispersed but interlinked nodes.

Sustained involvement and ownership. Just as short-term, albeit compassionate, outpourings of help after a major disaster such as the recent Indian Ocean tsunami do not sustain long-term development (Walker et al., 2005), launching the GHS with the sole purpose of helping to achieve the 5-year goals of PEPFAR will not solve the long-term health needs of PEPFAR countries and populations. However, the investments made by GHS participants and programs will contribute to those larger goals. Although the committee envisions the GHS as an ongoing activity of the U.S. government (thereby winning the trust of local stakeholders and ensuring some sustained involvement), it also envisions the GHS as adjusting to changing conditions over time, thereby allowing indigenous programs and personnel to take ownership of their own HIV/AIDS and other national health objectives.

THE GLOBAL HEALTH SERVICE AS STRATEGIC HUMANITARIANISM

Humanitarianism marks the recently augmented public health programs of many international organizations, including the United Nations, the World Bank, and the European Union, all of which have placed questions of public health on their agendas and joined in collective efforts against HIV/AIDS, TB, and malaria. Health is a complex concept with many varying historical, cultural, and social associations depending on its geographic and economic context. In western countries, a commitment to international health also has security-related motivations, especially with respect to the control of global epidemics. The recent energized global campaign against severe acute respiratory syndrome (SARS) and the mounting concern over a new global pandemic of avian influenza can certainly be seen in this light.

The GHS is proposed as a humanitarian program of the people of the United States at a time when the security of both PEPFAR countries and the United States is jeopardized by disease. In short, the GHS is a program of strategic humanitarianism. The committee believes that such a program will yield benefits in six key areas.

Humanitarian benefit. The GHS will enhance health in underserved areas and demonstrate the compassion of the American people.

Multicultural understanding. Like the U.S. Peace Corps, the GHS will foster relationships and multicultural understanding while mitigating anti-American sentiment overseas. It should also inspire a greater understanding of and commitment to global health on the part of the American people.

Collegial support and capacity building in affected countries. The emergence of HIV/AIDS has desperately worsened Africa's preexisting crisis in health manpower. Members and programs of the GHS will bring expertise, motivation, and muscle to long-term campaigns that might otherwise exhaust local human resources, despite enhanced access to new treatments. Their presence will also lead to the development of long-term cross-border personal networks.

Capacity building in the United States. The GHS will facilitate the development of new knowledge, experience, and public awareness, bolstering the ability of the United States to respond at home and abroad to many infectious/tropical disease threats resulting from globalization. Given the borderless nature of disease and the international and interdisciplinary nature of current scientific research, international collaborations are crucial to addressing global health issues. Epidemics such as SARS and HIV/AIDS, as well as physical disasters such as the recent tsunami in the Indian Ocean and earthquake in Iran, highlight the need for qualified professionals throughout the world to work together.

Countering of gender vulnerability. In many affected countries, legal, social, and economic factors have made girls and women especially vulnerable to the HIV/AIDS pandemic. In sub-Saharan Africa, girls and women represent 58 percent of those living with HIV/AIDS. In some of the worst-affected countries in southern Africa, intergenerational sex has led to HIV seroprevalence rates among girls aged 15 to 19 that are four to seven times higher than those among boys of the same age (Fleischman, 2003). In patrilineal African tribes, widows and children of victims of HIV/AIDS may also become destitute because the married couple's property reverts to the husband's family upon his death (LaFraniere, 2005). The GHS will combat gender vulnerability, especially through education and other AIDS prevention strategies.

Geopolitical security. HIV/AIDS will continue to be a destabilizing force in the world for decades to come. The infection is already eroding state capacity in sub-Saharan Africa (an important front in the war on terror), where 70 percent of currently infected patients reside. By 2010, 20 million children in Africa will have lost one or both parents to AIDS. Orphans and desocialized youth are especially vulnerable to exploitation in civil conflicts. Significant rates of HIV/AIDS in military populations also impact the ability of affected countries to safeguard their national interests and participate in regional peacekeeping. For this and other reasons, HIV/AIDS is a threat to regional, global, and U.S. security that merits major investments in human capital, as well as in drugs and technology.

REFERENCES

AAMC (Association of American Medical Colleges). 1984. *Medical School Graduation Questionnaire All Schools Report.* Washington, DC: AAMC.

AAMC. 2003. *Medical School Graduation Questionnaire All Schools Report.* Washington, DC: AAMC.

Fleischman J. 2003. *Fatal Vulnerabilities: Reducing the Acute Risk of HIV/AIDS Among Women and Girls.* Washington, DC: The CSIS Press.

LaFraniere S. 2005 (February 18). AIDS and custom leave African families nothing. *The New York Times.* A. A1.

Walker P, Wisner B, Leaning J, Minear L. 2005. Smoke and mirrors: Deficiencies in disaster funding. *British Medical Journal* 330:247–250.

5

Programs of the U.S. Global Health Service

This chapter describes six independent programs proposed for the Global Health Service (GHS). Each program would make a unique contribution to the mission of the GHS as discussed in Chapter 4; that is, to be flexible and responsive to target countries' needs for human resources for health to combat HIV/AIDS; to provide expertise in the form of caregivers, technical advisers, trainers, and mentors; and to sustain enduring relationships after U.S. health professionals work with colleagues on the ground. Taken together, the committee believes this set of programs can significantly augment human resource capacity in seeking to acheive the PEPFAR goals (see Chapter 1). The six programs are as follows:

- Global Health Service Corps
- Health Workforce Needs Assessment
- Fellowship Program
- Loan Repayment Program
- Twinning Program
- Clearinghouse

In brief, the committee envisions the Global Health Service Corps as the elite, anchor resource of the GHS, playing a far-reaching role in increasing the effectiveness of current in-country health personnel and expanding the future pool of resident health care assets. Corps members would serve for a minimum of 2 years overseas. The Fellowship and Loan Repayment Programs would provide incentives and reduce barriers to participation by qualified and motivated professionals serving for 1 and 2 years, respectively, overseas. The Twinning Program would mobilize health professionals for short- and long-term deployments keyed to specific needs of host countries and/or organizations. In addition, the committee proposes that gaps in human resources for health be evaluated for each PEPFAR focus country through formal needs assessments that could double as a baseline for follow-up evaluation of workforce capacity and distribution. Once these needs assessments had been carried out, uniform data for all countries could be compiled in a central electronic clearinghouse to enable the recruitment of other skilled health professionals. This virtual clearinghouse would thereby utilize information posting and global networking to further support the work of many other organizations and professionals contributing to the fight against global HIV/AIDS.

The committee believes that all six programs proposed for the GHS would be helpful in meeting the prevention, treatment, and care goals of PEPFAR. At the same time, some countries might choose to avail themselves of one resource more than another based on their individual needs.

The remainder of this chapter is divided into six sections, each describing one of the six proposed GHS programs (for a summary, see Table 5-1). Each section presents in turn background information (often echoing themes and evidence presented earlier in this report), the committee's recommendation for that program, a fuller description of the program, and the rationale and evidence behind the committee's recommendation. In some cases, there is also a discussion of deployment, public versus private placement of the program, and program costs.

TABLE 5-1 Six Proposed Programs of the U.S. Global Health Service

Global Health Service Corps	A small group of highly skilled professionals, deployed for a minimum of 2 years
Health Workforce Needs Assessment	A standardized health personnel needs assessment for all PEPFAR focus countries
Fellowship Program	A $35,000 award to enable health professionals to work overseas for a minimum of 1 year
Loan Repayment Program	A $25,000 loan repayment for qualified health professionals for each year of a 2-year service overseas
Twinning Program	A mechanism for short-, medium-, or long-term mobilization of needed skilled professionals
Clearinghouse	A resource using information technology for recruitment, information posting, and networking

GLOBAL HEALTH SERVICE CORPS

If the PEPFAR goals are to be achieved, HIV/AIDS prevention and treatment programs will likely need cadres of health personnel far larger than those currently available in most PEPFAR focus countries (USAID, 2003; USAID Guyana, 2003; WHO, 2003). In addition, the rapid scale-up of antiretroviral therapy (ART) will require expertise and knowledge in a variety of medical and nonmedical areas often unavailable in resource-constrained settings. Indeed, as discussed earlier, there is broad recognition that the limited stock of health workers in many of the PEPFAR focus countries alone could spell failure for the scale-up effort (Kober and Van Damme, 2004). Factors contributing to profound shortages of health workers in these countries are limited baseline educational capacity; the active emigration of many newly trained health personnel; low pay and morale, poor working conditions, and inadequate management, encouraging the departure of health workers; movement of other workers to the private sector; and HIV/AIDS-related attrition of existing staff (WHO, 2004). Additional problems at the health services delivery level include not only shortages and poor distribution of doctors and nurses, but also weak program management, poor technical support, inadequate supplies of drugs, and lack of equipment and infrastructure (HLF, 2004; WHO, 2004). In sum, inadequacies of both health care delivery and infrastructure pose extraordinary challenges to building a sustainable workforce.

To address the critical need in all PEPFAR focus countries for key specialized health, management, and technical professionals, the committee proposes the establishment of a Global Health Service Corps. This cadre of specialists would be available to assist with and support the implementation of national strategic HIV/AIDS programs. Its members would work in such areas as medical and nursing education, information technology for health systems, health systems design and management, and laboratory and pharmaceutical management. The common purpose of the Corps would be to enhance the effectiveness of current health personnel and support efforts to expand the health workforce of the future. Thus, the Corps would play a key role in the GHS's overall contribution to the successful realization of PEPFAR goals.

Recommendation 3: *Establish a U.S. Global Health Service Corps to send key health personnel to PEPFAR countries on a full-time/long-term basis.* The committee recommends the establishment of a full-salaried/long-term U.S. Global Health Service Corps for the recruitment, placement, and support of U.S. health, technical, and management professionals in PEPFAR countries. Because of the critical and highly visible nature of this Corps and the necessity for it to coordinate closely with PEPFAR, the committee further recommends that it be established and administered as a program of the federal government. U.S. Global Health Service Corps professionals should be selected and deployed based on the prioritized needs identified by ministries of health in conjunction with in-country PEPFAR teams. Assignments will be made for a minimum of 2 years with placements in areas and programs where Corps members' presence would have maximum impact on enhancing the human capacity to prevent and treat HIV/AIDS. The committee proposes an initial deployment of 150 U.S. Global Health Service Corps professionals in the 15 PEPFAR countries based on needs assessment, placement development, and the availability of professionals with the required skills.

Program Description

Structure

The Global Health Service Corps could be established as a program of the federal government. This strategic positioning of the program would allow coordination of the Corps' mission with the PEPFAR program and U.S. government country teams both abroad and domestically.

As the committee envisions the Corps, health professionals, as well as experts in management and technical matters related to health, would be dispatched for extended periods of service to PEPFAR focus countries. The primary purpose of these placements would be to advance the PEPFAR goals by assigning highly qualified personnel to key positions in newly expanding national programs of HIV/AIDS prevention and treatment. The Corps' specialized professionals would be deployed on a full-time basis for a minimum of 2 years to provide technical assistance for scale-up of these programs. Given the heterogeneous needs of the 15 PEPFAR focus countries, the Corps should encompass a similarly diverse range of expertise, from clinicians and clinician trainers to experts in such nonclinical areas as information technology, health systems management, and laboratory and pharmaceutical management. Deployed U.S. professionals would be expected to work side-by-side with their host country counterparts to maximize the transfer of their skills and to help to develop the next generation of local health leadership. Priority would be given to positions and roles with the greatest potential to have a multiplier effect in promoting indigenous skills and capacity.

The Global Health Service Corps would also play a meaningful role in the United States. It would become a dedicated program of the U.S. government supporting the long-term service of personnel in global health. It would provide career options for U.S. health, management, and technical professionals committed to addressing the HIV/AIDS pandemic and other global scourges. As such, the Corps could become an enduring instrument of U.S. foreign aid, foreign policy, and health policy.

Eligibility and Selection Process

The Global Health Service Corps would work in close coordination with PEPFAR; U.S. government in-country teams; and current governmental efforts to scale up HIV/AIDS prevention and treatment programs abroad, including those of the U.S. Agency for International Development (USAID), the Centers for Disease Control and Prevention (CDC), and the Health Resources and Services Administration (HRSA). The Corps could recruit commissioned officers of the U.S. Public Health Service and civil service professionals currently in government service, as well as nongovernmental professionals, into its ranks. It would call on reserved and retired commissioned officers and attract specialists from the private sector, universities, and industry. It would use the Intergovernmental Personnel Act (see Box 5-1) and the GHS Loan Repayment program (described later in this chapter) to assist in its recruitment efforts.

The development and prioritization of positions within the Corps would be the responsibility of PEPFAR country teams in conjunction with the respective ministries of health. Using the results of the workforce needs assessments discussed in the next section, these PEPFAR/ministry of health teams would identify key country-level clinical, management, and technical workforce needs associated with the PEPFAR mission. Requests to address these needs with Corps personnel would be made to the Corps, and assignments would be made based on prioritization of needs and identification and availability of appropriate professionals. Priority in making assignments would be given to those supporting the infrastructure development and sustainability of national HIV/AIDS programs. In all cases, the assignments should be relevant to long-term capacity building in the country and should, to the extent possible, involve the transfer of skills to host country professionals.

Deployment

Individual Corps members would be deployed abroad as government employees with all associated benefits. Following admission into the Corps, members would undergo a country-specific orientation in the United States, followed by a site-specific orientation in the country of assignment. Regardless of previous experience, all Corps members will need to acquire familiarity with cultural and ethical issues specific to their countries of assignment, as well as the particulars of their job. Corps members would generally be supervised by their PEPFAR country team while also being integrated to

---

BOX 5-1
The Intergovernmental Personnel Act

The Intergovernmental Personnel Act (IPA) Mobility Program provides for the temporary assignment of personnel to facilitate cooperation between the federal government and state and local governments, colleges and universities, Indian tribal governments, federally funded research and development centers, and other eligible organizations. The goal of the program is to facilitate the movement of employees for short periods of time to serve a sound public purpose.

Typically, only senior executive–level positions are filled by an IPA agreement. The assignment is for 2 years, extendable for an additional 2 years. The recipient of the appointment continues to be paid by his or her parent organization at full salary and benefits, and the parent organization receives a negotiated reimbursement from the government.

At American University for example, Interagency Personnel Agreement (IPA) assignments provide opportunities for faculty members to work for the federal government on special assignment. These assignments require a contract between the university and the employing agency, and must be processed through the Office of Sponsored Programs (OSP).

While on an IPA, the faculty member is "on detail" to the agency (or office) while still on active service at the university. Many faculty members have been able to combine an IPA with their sabbaticals and thus arrange a full-year leave at full pay.

Most IPAs are for a full-time commitment, although arrangements for a partial IPA may be approved, depending on the nature of the IPA assignment, if the time committed to university service is substantial. The university does not charge indirect costs on IPAs, however, the university does not provide cost share on such agreements either.

Sources: http://www.american.edu/academics/provost/dean/faculty/leave_policy.htm.

---

the extent possible into the host country organization to which they are assigned. In addition, coordination and cooperation would be encouraged among Corps personnel in a given country and between these personnel and local public health authorities. Given the complexity and importance of the anticipated assignments and the need for strong collegial relationships to develop, tours of duty should be at least 2 years in length. Assignments might be extended when there is agreement on doing so among Corps leadership, the host organization, and the Corps member. Corps members could serve sequential assignments in different countries depending on skills needed, prioritization, and availability. Evaluation of all assignments would be carried out on an annual basis.

The committee believes that the Global Health Service Corps should be launched modestly, but that it should also be large enough to establish its identity, make a contribution, and garner experience. An initial deployment of 150 Corps members (prorated according to need and availability) would achieve these aims while allowing the Corps to remain manageable as a new enterprise.

Rationale and Evidence

Why a Global Health Service Corps?

As discussed throughout this report, a lack of skilled and trained health professionals is one of the principal barriers to the rapid scale-up of HIV/ AIDS prevention and treatment programs in the PEPFAR focus countries (Adano et al., 2004; Wyss, 2004a,b). A range of skills is needed, particularly at the level of key clinical, management, and technical leadership positions essential to building the infrastructure of HIV/AIDS treatment systems (WHO, 2002). Because of the specialized nature of these positions and the long-term requirements of the work, volunteer health professionals and those with short-term availability will be of limited utility in addressing core country-level needs. It will be the role of the Global Health Service Corps, working with public health leaders in the PEPFAR focus countries, to provide specialized health personnel for extended assignments to fill these positions and accelerate program scale-up.

The production of new health care workers has not kept pace with the growing demand for greater workforce capacity (RATN, 2003). There is a shortage of trained workers with specific experience in the clinical management of HIV/AIDS treatment programs; there are also severe shortages of well-trained professionals needed to handle other critical functions, such as commodity logistics, pharmaceutical regulation, information management for laboratory support, and operations research (Interim Pharmacy Council of South Africa, 1998; IOM, 2005; Katerere and Matowe, 2003; Ntuli et al., 2003). Uganda illustrates this point. One of the primary constraints on increasing Ugandan ART enrolees from 25,500 to 60,000 by the end of 2005 is the lack of qualified health staff. Most likely, the target will not be reached unless an aggressive intervention is quickly developed and implemented (Adano et al., 2004), yet the country faces an imposing challenge in producing the needed professionals (see below). Kenya also appears to be facing human resource shortage issues. In addition to dealing with the greater numbers of patients due to the upward-spiralling HIV epidemic, Kenyan health workers treating patients with AIDS and AIDS-related illnesses have found that the complexity of the disease poses new demands (Personal communication, Annalisa Trama, UNAIDS Kenya, December 1, 2004). Many such patients require full-time attention and longer hospital stays. As a result, roughly half of the patients in Kenyan medical wards have AIDS-related illnesses.

A low stock of skilled health workers is not the only impediment to scale-up; fragmentation of the employment process also plays a role (HLF, 2004). Country-level planning and human resource management capacity are often limited in developing countries and inadequately responsive to the changing priorities likely as more people begin ART or receive prevention counselling. An important structural problem in some areas is the undue centralization of government health systems. When all budget and policy decisions are made by the central government, a sense of powerlessness and lack of accountability can result at the district and province levels where the services are delivered (Personal communication, Stephen Moore, CDC-Nairobi, October 24, 2004).

The challenge of producing skilled health care workers in the PEPFAR countries is illustrated by Uganda. Although educational institutions (medical schools, nursing schools, schools for health science) produce personnel who then serve as trained professional staff, the country is not generating enough doctors, nurses, pharmacists, or laboratory technologists to run basic health services, let alone HIV/AIDS-specific services (Adano et al., 2004). In addition, many recent graduates of health training institutions cannot find employment because of budget constraints and restrictions on personnel recruitment. Some cadres of trained health workers feel underutilized because they cannot obtain jobs in their areas of professional training that will maximize their potential and create opportunities for professional growth. This lack of career paths and motivation among young professionals has long-term consequences for human resource planning.

Costs

Salaries, benefits, and travel would account for most of the costs of the Global Health Service Corps. Projecting the exact cost of the Corps is not possible without making a series of assumptions about the personnel system to be used, the disciplines and seniority of the personnel involved, and the details of the approaches to orientation and supervision to be used for the Corps. A reasonable estimate of costs for the Corps can be derived from CDC, which deploys health professionals abroad using government personnel systems; its rough estimate for sending a skilled professional overseas is $250,000 per year per person.[1] Using this yardstick, the deployment of an

---

[1]The total can be $300,000 or more depending on certain factors, such as whether the country is more expensive; the base salary is higher (e.g., a medical epidemiologist compared with a junior administrator); how many children the person has (the government pays school fees at $10,000–15,000 per child per year); whether the total tour is shorter (because the costs of the move and set-up [e.g., housing] are amortized over fewer years); or security-related costs are increased (Personal Communication, Michael St. Louis, CDC, February 23, 2005).

initial Corps of 150 individuals as recommended by the committee would require a budget of $37.5 million (150 × $250,000).

The committee discussed these costs at length, appreciating that the investment required for a fully salaried, full-time/long-term professional would be substantial, and that many other health-related goods and services could be purchased for the same sum. On balance, however, the committee concluded that the investment in a small and specialized Corps that would play a pivotal role in ART scale-up and global health development is an equally important commitment on the part of PEPFAR and the United States. The committee notes further that a $37.5 million aggregate yearly investment represents approximately 1 percent of the current annual PEPFAR budget.

Options for Placement

Public versus Private Sector

Several options exist for the organization and placement of the Global Health Service Corps as the anchor program of the GHS. The first decision to be made is whether to locate the Corps in the public or private sector. The committee decided that all the programs of the GHS should be managed in a unitary fashion within the federal government, while individual programs might be candidates for public–private collaboration or placement in the private sector through contract mechanisms (see Chapter 4).

The committee believes strongly that the specialized nature of the Corps, its requirement for long-term service, its visibility, and its potential to be the signature program of the U.S. global health effort argue for its being established as a program of the federal government. Doing so would address important and sensitive issues, including the need for close coordination with PEPFAR and other U.S. global health and foreign policy initiatives. The committee discussed at length the option of placing the Corps in the private sector, managed through a federal government contract. The committee members were aware of many not-for-profit and for-profit organizations under government contract that have been successful in deploying health professionals abroad. These contracts are usually framed in terms of the delivery of specific services and recruitment of health professionals as assets to help to achieve the goals of the contract. Private firms working in this area are generally credited with the ability to locate health professionals and move them into the field quickly. However, working at the government-to-government level is an area in which private firms are less well positioned. For this reason, the committee believes the Corps would better be established as a program of the U.S. government, and that such federal placement would best serve recruitment, placement, mission coordination, skill banking, retention, and long-term program development. A federally based Corps would also greatly facilitate the program's integration with PEPFAR and in-country strategies.

Multiple agencies and individuals—including the American Medical Student Association, United Methodist Committee on Relief, International Health Medical Education Consortium, and American Society for Tropical Medicine—testified to the committee regarding the growing interest in careers in global health. This interest is seen across the career spectrum—students, established experts, and health professionals wanting to retire early to participate in health programs abroad (Kelly, 2004; Palmer, 2004; Weaver, 2004). The committee believes strongly that this interest should be captured by the range of programs envisioned for the GHS, but that the Corps in particular should provide deployment opportunities and model careers in global health. As the signature program of the GHS initiative, the Corps should be a program of the federal government that will make a statement at home and abroad about the importance of careers in global health and the commitment of the U.S. government to the long-term mission of improving health worldwide. Moreover, a federal Corps would be in a position to recruit from the ranks of the Public Health Service and civil service while also recruiting new professionals into its ranks.

Potential Federal Agencies

A number of agencies of the U.S. government that currently deploy health professionals should be considered in deciding about the positioning of the Global Health Service Corps. Each is briefly discussed below; a listing of these agencies' attributes that may be helpful in making this decision is provided in Appendix G. Moreover, the experience of these agencies should inform policy makers designing the Corps.

The Peace Corps. The Peace Corps is well established, well recognized, and well regarded with respect to the placement of U.S. citizens abroad. Over the years, public health has been among its areas of focus. The Peace Corps, however, functions with volunteers and does not provide recompense likely to appeal to many senior-level clinical, technical, or management personnel undertaking extended assignments. Rather, the Peace Corps provides volunteers with a living allowance that enables them to live in a manner similar to that of the local people in their community (United States Peace Corps, 2005a).

Centers for Disease Control and Prevention. CDC has had extensive experience with foreign assignments. Through its Global AIDS program, it has roughly 40 direct hires in the PEPFAR focus countries, with an average of

2 to 3 per country (CDC, 2005). CDC has a strong epidemiologic tradition (the Epidemic Intelligence Service in particular) and is very well recognized in public health circles worldwide. Its expertise, however, is largely in surveillance and prevention; it has less experience and less of a mandate regarding health systems development or the personnel needed to assist in such efforts.

National Health Service Corps. The National Health Service Corps (NHSC) has almost 35 years of experience with the placement of health professionals in underserved areas and with scholarship and loan repayment programs as recruitment strategies (NHSC, 2003). It has an identity that is mission driven and easily equates with a domestic version of the proposed Global Health Service Corps. However, NHSC has no international mandate or experience, and its program is limited to clinicians.

Indian Health Service. The Indian Health Service (IHS) is an agency within the Department of Health and Human Services. It provides health services to approximately 1.5 million American Indians and Alaska Natives who belong to more than 557 federally recognized tribes in 35 states. Similar to the proposed GHS, the IHS has a recruitment website, administers scholarship and loan repayment programs, employs a variety of health professionals, and encourages commissioned officers to participate (IHS, 2005). The IHS does not work internationally, however, and has a broad focus on general health care not specific to HIV/AIDS.

Other agencies of the federal government also send health professionals abroad. USAID employs multiple contract mechanisms to sponsor health programs that deploy U.S. health personnel; HRSA oversees similar deployments on a smaller scale and targeted to the PEPFAR focus countries. Likewise, the U.S. Armed Forces deploy large numbers of health personnel abroad, both in support of the military mission and in humanitarian relief efforts.

The experience of all of the above U.S. government agencies should be taken into account when considering the placement of the Global Health Service Corps. After examining the various options, the committee concluded that the effectiveness, identity, and mission of the Corps to support the PEPFAR goals would best be served by the establishment of a discrete program of the federal government managed by the GHS. Furthermore, the structure of the Corps would then be in place and prepared to mobilize health personnel proactively for emerging global health crises in the future.

HEALTH WORKFORCE NEEDS ASSESSMENT

Timely and accurate information on workforce needs will be essential to maximize the impact of programs mobilizing health personnel to achieve the PEPFAR goals. Despite the key role of human resources in the functioning of health systems, few well-conducted qualitative or quantitative studies have assessed the adequacy of the health care workforce in the PEPFAR focus countries (SWEF Research Network, 2005). Failing to complete such an assessment before initiating a scale-up plan for health personnel could ultimately undermine the effectiveness of the initiative. Access to systematic data on vacancies in the health workforce would also provide valuable information for individuals and institutions engaged in mobilizing health professionals for service in the PEPFAR focus countries.

According to a critical review performed for the committee (see Appendix C), the PEPFAR focus countries need better data to project the quantity of health care workers needed to scale up HIV/AIDS activities. Better data are also needed to establish the existing skill mix of providers and other support staff in each country, as well as the distribution of workers in urban versus rural settings and the public versus private health sector. In estimating national stocks, worker profiles, and the distribution of personnel, moreover, certain assumptions regarding the service delivery model must be made. For example, the annual growth rate of human resource stock over the next 5 years is assumed to be equivalent to the annual growth rate of the past 5 years—4.5 percent according to the available data. Other assumptions relate to the numbers of patients and diagnosis rates of HIV infection. Despite these limitations, estimates of human resource needs have been made for the PEPFAR focus countries, some of which are presented in this chapter.

Collated data from a thorough workforce needs assessment not only would inform host and donor countries about where and how assistance would most effectively build human resource capacity to achieve the PEPFAR goals, but also could serve as a baseline for follow-up evaluation of national health capacity. Finally, although HIV/AIDS is the target of funding for the PEPFAR program, the inseparability of this infection from tuberculosis (TB) and malaria in most of the 15 focus countries should be recognized (see Chapter 2). A comprehensive needs assessment would take into account the overlap in the work of doctors combating all three diseases.

Recommendation 4: *Undertake a uniform health workforce needs assessment.* **The committee recommends that the PEPFAR country teams, in collaboration with ministries of health, initiate assessments of in-country requirements for health personnel to achieve PEPFAR goals. These assessments should form the basis for national human resources for health plans. These assessments would also generate a valuable**

baseline inventory for all mobilization programs and subsequent evaluation activities. The data from all countries should be collected in a standardized fashion, updated regularly, and maintained in the electronic database of the U.S. Global Health Service Clearinghouse "Opportunity Bank," available to professionals interested in service in PEPFAR countries. Timely and accurate information on workforce needs will be essential to maximize the impact of programs designed to mobilize health personnel to achieve PEPFAR goals. Current national needs assessments are irregular, nonstandardized, and not available at any single site. Local placement strategies and global recruitment efforts would be greatly strengthened by a regularized needs assessment and dissemination initiative.

Program Description

A standardized health workforce needs assessment is necessary for all the PEPFAR focus countries. Responsibility for leadership of this effort should lie with each country's ministry of health in conjunction with the PEPFAR in-country program. With adequate training and staffing, ministries could perform their own data collection and analysis using this assessment. In countries where the ministry of health is not able to perform its own assessment, employing an outside organization may be necessary; a not-for-profit organization or private company experienced in analyzing human resources for ART scale-up in developing countries could conduct the assessment and analyze the data. A likely result of these assessments will be the identification of methods—such as those described in this report—for strengthening the human resource capacity of ministries of health to monitor and evaluate their programs.

Tools are currently available to assist NGOs and countries in conducting human resource management needs assessments for HIV/AIDS environments (MSH, 2003); human resource development assessments (MSH, 1998); rapid assessments of human resources for health (WHO, 2004); and baseline assessment tools for preventing mother-to-child transmission of HIV (FHI, 2003). A compilation of the most salient measurements collected from these and other previously developed assessment instruments would be a most effective means of analyzing country needs with regard to the goals of PEPFAR. However, it is important to note that unless ministries of health see the value, have the capacity, and commit to the process, these tools may not be used and/or updated appropriately.

The instrument employed for workforce needs assessment must be uniform for all countries so the data can be logged, shared, and used for resource allocation purposes in a standardized fashion. The results would assist PEPFAR in determining the numbers and types of positions needing support in various countries through the GHS programs. Personnel needs identified in this fashion would also be available for posting in the GHS Clearinghouse Opportunities Bank (see below) in a systematic manner. These openings could potentially be filled by U.S. professionals seeking jobs overseas, and continuous follow-up measurements would provide tracking of open positions. Additionally, the initial assessment could serve as a baseline for follow-up analyses of human resources in HIV/AIDS health systems.

Rationale and Evidence

The GHS would be responsible for sending U.S. health and other professionals to countries that expressed a substantiated need for a particular form of assistance. Conducting a workforce needs assessment is an essential first step in establishing and verifying such needs (MSH, 2004). Currently, there is no uniformity in the way PEPFAR countries collect and analyze data on their human resources for health. This variability is a major impediment to the fair and equitable distribution of workforce resources among the 15 PEPFAR focus countries. Lack of consistency among countries in how human resource development strategies are monitored and evaluated on an international basis has also been noted (Diallo et al., 2003). Although all of the focus countries have country strategic plans through USAID, these plans were not designed to address human resource issues and are therefore not useful in this regard. Country plans drafted by U.S. government teams in each PEPFAR focus country were not available for review at the time of this writing.

A review of the few available HIV/AIDS-related workforce needs assessments (listed in Table 5-2) reveals that some countries have already taken the initiative to address their workforce requirements for ART scale-up. Each assessment provides valuable information, but none of them considers all aspects of current and future workforce needs for accomplishing the PEPFAR goals. One possible exception is *The Zambia HIV/AIDS Workforce Study: Preparing for Scale-Up*—a comprehensive analysis that addresses whether Zambia will have the staff to scale up prevention of mother-to-child transmission and ART to reach its targeted number of clients (Huddart et al., 2004). The Ugandan and South African reports also cover many workforce issues and project staffing needs for a wide variety of health workers in addition to doctors, nurses, and pharmacists (Adano et al., 2004; South Africa Ministry of Health, 2003).

Despite a concerted effort, the committee was unable to locate an appropriate health workforce needs assessment addressing all of PEPFAR's activities and targets. The commissioned paper presented in Appendix C is

TABLE 5-2 Workforce Needs Assessments for PEPFAR Focus Countries

Country/Region	Assessment
Uganda	*Rapid Assessment of the Human Resource Implications of Scaling Up HIV/AIDS Services in Uganda* (Adano et al., 2004)
Zambia	*The Zambia HIV/AIDS Workforce Study: Preparing for Scale-Up* (Huddart et al., 2004)
South Africa	*Operational Plan for Comprehensive HIV and AIDS Care, Management and Treatment for South Africa* (South Africa Ministry of Health, 2003)
Nigeria	*Scaling Up Antiretroviral Treatment in the Public Sector in Nigeria* (Kombe et al., 2004); and *Nigeria: Rapid Assessment of HIV/AIDS Care in the Public and Private Sectors* (PHRplus, 2004)
Eastern and Southern Africa	*Eastern and Southern Africa Regional HIV/AIDS Training Needs Assessment* (RATN, 2003)
Sub-Saharan Africa	*Scaling-up Antiretroviral Treatment and Human Resources for Health* (Wyss, 2004a)

an attempt to estimate these needs, although several limitations of data availability hamper its precision. On the basis of available data, it appears that the total human resource stock delivering all health services in 2004 in the PEPFAR focus countries was 566,580 (74 percent nurses, 21 percent doctors, and 5 percent pharmacists). Applying these 2004 baseline data and assuming that existing conditions will not change, the total number of health workers is projected to increase to 592,076 by 2008, an annual growth rate of approximately 4.5 percent. This increase is driven primarily by Nigeria, South Africa, and Vietnam, all countries with large populations and high personnel totals. Meanwhile, countries such as Tanzania and Uganda will see a decrease in their total human resource stock. The remaining 10 PEPFAR countries will see minimum growth in their health workforce in the next 4 years.

The number of health workers needed to achieve the PEPFAR goals—not including laboratory technicians, social workers, counselors, and community health workers—was approximately 11,200 in 2004 and will be roughly 56,000 by 2008 because of the planned scale-up of the PEPFAR program. These are broad estimates for all 15 focus countries. The actual needs vary from country to country, with greatest human resource gaps existing in those countries with the greatest HIV prevalence rates.

Projected gaps in trained HIV/AIDS personnel suggest a great need for master trainers to train health workers in HIV/AIDS care. The approximate number of master trainers needed so that the 15 PEPFAR focus countries can provide full HIV/AIDS services to all eligible patients is 3,000—1,100 doctors, 1,200 nurses, and 700 pharmacists. To reach the PEPFAR goals by 2008, roughly 1,600 master trainers will be needed.

Given the data limitations described above, there is a clear and compelling need for the proposed health care workforce assessment. Better data on health care workforce needs obtained through the proposed assessment would also assist countries in determining the allocation of their resources. In addition, it is important to evaluate overall health systems capacity when scaling up HIV/AIDS prevention, treatment, and care services; indeed, many countries have begun such an effort to varying degrees.

FELLOWSHIP PROGRAM

As discussed earlier, many health professionals in the United States are eager to volunteer in the developing world. In fact, the International Medical Volunteers Association (IMVA) currently has a registry of more than 5,300 health professionals, many of whom are U.S. citizens, seeking overseas medical assignments (IMVA, 2005). International volunteer activities available to health professionals have traditionally been initiated and supervised by academic centers, NGOs, faith-based organizations, hospitals, and other charitable organizations. The *Journal of the American Medical Association* publishes an inventory entitled "Physicians Service Opportunities Abroad" every 3 years that lists more than 60 organizations offering a variety of short-term volunteer opportunities for health professionals (Vastag, 2002). However, many interested candidates are unable to overcome the financial or logistical barriers to significant periods of overseas service. As a result, they have had little or no impact upon human resource needs in sub-Saharan Africa. The proposed GHS Fellowship Program would provide incentives and reduce barriers to mobilize a broad range of trained professionals with skills relevant to addressing the human resource crisis in the PEPFAR focus countries. GHS Fellowships would enable awardees already paired with a host organization to commit a meaningful period of service to a PEPFAR country and participate in direct patient care, systems development, training of trainers, and scaling up of resources and capacities to respond to the HIV/AIDS crisis.

Recommendation 5: *Create a U.S. Global Health Service Fellowship Program.* **The committee recommends the creation of a U.S. Global Health Service Fellowship Program that would provide professional recognition and a $35,000 award to qualified U.S. personnel to enable**

commitment to programs of service in **PEPFAR countries.** This competitive program would fund a prestigious award to individuals willing to make medium-term commitments of 1 year or longer to provide health care, training, and technical assistance in countries in need. It would provide career-long recognition as well as immediate financial assistance.

Program Description

Structure

The GHS Fellowship Program is designed to provide qualified health personnel wishing to work abroad with incentives to serve within the framework of the PEPFAR mission. The structure of the program would engage professionals by reducing financial and logistical barriers to service, while also focusing their activities to align with the PEPFAR goals. Much like the prestigious Fulbright awards, the GHS Fellowships would confer honor and professional recognition on their recipients.

The GHS Fellowship program would be housed together with the other programs of the GHS. The implementing agency would have oversight and management responsibilities, and a national board made up of experts in the field would oversee the direction and mission of the program. An annual award in the amount of $35,000 would not be meant to cover all expenses, but to supplement the recipient's other financial resources and assist with travel expenses and the cost of living. Participants would also be eligible to apply for the GHS Loan Repayment Program (see below).

Fellows would be required to serve for a minimum of 1 year, and their work would be focused on specific projects structured in collaboration with a host organization. This close collaboration would minimize the amount of time required for recipients to adjust to their new work environment and begin the tasks at hand. The program would start small but grow quickly. One hundred awards would be made in the first year (roughly 5–10 per country, prorated by need) increasing to 1,000 awards by the third year of the program. Placement would respond to the needs of the PEPFAR focus countries as defined by each country operating plan and the Opportunity Bank of the GHS Clearinghouse (discussed later in this chapter).

Eligibility and Selection Process

As is true for many prestigious awards, there would be a competitive process leading to participation in the GHS Fellowship Program. U.S. citizenship or permanent resident status would be an initial requirement; in addition, applicants would have to be trained professionals, including but not limited to nurses, doctors, midwives, laboratory workers, data managers, HIV trainers, pharmacists, social scientists, and health care professionals with experience relevant to the HIV/AIDS mission of PEPFAR. To apply for the award, applicants would have to have a preidentified health services or health systems destination in a PEPFAR focus country. This destination would have to be documented, and the applicant would have to have the full support of the host organization in writing. This process would allow the applicant to select and design a suitable position that would be aligned with the needs of the host country.

The purpose of this award would be to build quality care and human capacity in resource-constrained settings; proposed positions should therefore reflect this goal. Applicants proposing basic research projects would not be accepted. The committee acknowledges that operations research may be needed in some settings and organizations to identify better or more efficient ways of administering HIV/AIDS prevention, treatment, and care; depending on local needs, such research could be considered as an aspect of a project.

To apply, an individual would first submit a work plan, requisite credentials, references, and a statement of commitment from a host organization either working or based in a PEPFAR focus country. A selection panel comprising health professionals from the United States and focus countries would then review the application and score the applicant using a uniform measure. Points would be awarded for experience and level of expertise, as well as quality of references and work plan. Points for alignment with PEPFAR and national priorities would be added to the individual scores to create composite scores that would ultimately be used to rank order candidates and make the awards.

Deployment

GHS fellows would receive country-specific cultural and ethical training both before departure and upon arrival on site. In addition to receiving a packet of written information, fellows would be referred to the GHS Clearinghouse, where they would find country-specific information. Upon arrival on site, they would undergo intensive orientation organized in cooperation with the host organization. If a common foreign language (such as French, Spanish, or Portuguese) were required, the fellow would be expected to be fluent in that language before arrival. Local language training could be provided if applicable. Predeparture orientation would also include information about health needs, such as immunizations, malaria prophylaxis, and reliable sources of evacuation and health insurance. Health insurance would be required for all fellows serving overseas. Information about medical licensure, although available through the Clearinghouse, would also be provided to the participant.

Evaluation

Evaluation of the GHS Fellowship Program would take place on many levels. A participatory evaluation of the field work and experience should include the host organization, the agency granting the award, and the fellow. This evaluation should include such information as the number of professionals trained, the number of patients treated, and the satisfaction level of the host organization with the services provided by the fellow. The infrastructure of the host organization should be assessed to ensure that it does not become overburdened with volunteers. A second evaluation would be an exit survey, completed by each fellow. The results would inform the selection committee about the usefulness of the fellow's plan, whether the plan could be replicated in other areas, and other valuable lessons learned by the returning fellow. The data compiled from these exit surveys would be collected and made accessible to future fellows via electronic dissemination.

Rationale and Evidence

Why a Fellowship Program?

The shortage and uneven distribution of health workers has been discussed at length in previous chapters as the primary constraint on achieving the PEPFAR goals. Many existing academic and government fellowship programs in the United States send professionals abroad whose main focus is HIV research. For example, the Fogarty International Center at the National Institutes of Health has forged global relationships focused on research through the AIDS International Training and Research Program. The program provides HIV/AIDS-related research training to strengthen the capacity of institutions in low- and middle-income countries (Fogarty International Center, 2002). Multidisciplinary training is offered to physicians, dentists, pharmacists, scientists, and support personnel from selected developing countries. The training emphasizes research methods relevant to epidemiologic and behavioral studies related to AIDS, HIV transmission, and treatment to prevent or delay morbidity and mortality in HIV-infected persons. However, the committee could find no fellowship program focused on training counselors, providing care, or assisting in the skilled management of ART scale-up. The many U.S. health care workers who go overseas for clinical work do so either through short-term placements under travel fellowships from medical schools, medical societies, or nongovernmental organizations (NGOs) such as Doctors without Borders, or as volunteers with charitable or faith-based organizations (Vastag, 2002). Few of these clinical programs offer any long-term legacy or sustainability within a country. A 1-year GHS Fellowship would serve as an innovative incentive to mobilize large numbers of volunteer U.S. professionals rapidly for a meaningful time period to the PEPFAR focus countries in support of the PEPFAR goals. Moreover, this program could ultimately strengthen long-term ties among professionals working to fight HIV/AIDS globally and become a model program for responding to future emerging global health crises.

Program Design

In developing the concept of the GHS Fellowship Program, the committee was guided by various models discussed in this report. Just as the Fulbright awards represent opportunities for collaboration in global education, the Fogarty International Center opportunities for research, and the Peace Corps opportunities for diplomacy and cross-cultural exchange, the GHS Fellowship Program would offer opportunities for partnering in global health.

Selection of Fellows. The GHS Fellowship Program is meant to be selective and competitive, and the point system described above would allow only the most qualified professionals to receive awards. The point system would also ensure the awarding of fellowships to applicants who most closely meet the needs of a specific country. The selection process for the GHS Fellowship Program was modeled on that of the Traditional Fulbright Scholar Program, which has eligibility criteria including U.S. citizenship, a Ph.D. or equivalent professional/terminal degree (for professionals outside of academia, recognized professional standing and substantial professional accomplishments), relevant experience that corresponds to the level of work in the field, foreign language proficiency as necessary, and sound physical and mental health (CIES, 2005). Since its inception in 1946, the Fulbright program has provided more than 255,000 participants the opportunity to study and teach in each other's countries. The program awards about 4,500 grants a year, and its alumni include Nobel and Pulitzer Prize winners, ambassadors, governors, senators, artists, prime ministers and heads of state, professors, scientists, Supreme Court justices, and many others (CIES, 2005).

Number of Fellows. As noted above, the committee agreed that the Fellowship Program should start with 100 awards in the first year (about 6 per country, prorated by need), increasing to 1,000 awards by the third year of the program. Starting small would allow the infrastructure of the program to develop and would enable feedback from the first set of fellows to be incorporated into the program. The proposal to scale up to 1,000 volunteers per year is based on the fact that the Peace Corps deploys around 4,000 volunteers per year (Rieffel, 2003). As of September 2004, the Peace Corps had 7,733 volunteers abroad, 20 percent of whom (1,546) worked in the health sector. With the advent of PEPFAR in 2003, the Peace Corps[2] committed more than 1,000 new volunteers to work on HIV/AIDS education, but still has not made meaningful inroads in meeting human resource needs (IOM, 2005; United States Peace Corps, 2005a). Similarly for comparison, the IHS employs 900 doctors (out of a total workforce of 15,000), who provide health services to approximately 1.5 million American Indians and Alaska Natives in 35 states (IHS, 2005). Assuming that IHS doctors make at least the median salary for a GS-15 employee in 2005 ($103,071), this program spends more than $92,700,000 each year on doctors alone (OPM, 2005a).

The committee recommends that the GHS Fellowship Program start small with 5–10 participants in 15 countries in order to pilot the program's infrastructure. At the level of awards envisioned, the cost of the program would start at $3.5 million ($35,000 × 100 awards) and grow to $35 million ($35,000 × 1,000 awards) by the third year of the program, representing about 0.1 percent of the current PEPFAR budget and 1 percent of the projected PEPFAR budget, respectively.

Compensation. After reviewing the literature, the committee decided that the amount of $35,000 would be reasonable to assist fellows with living expenses. According to JHPIEGO, the cost of sustaining a health professional with no salary implications for 1 year ranges from $32,994 in Zambia to $45,832 in Kenya.[3] It costs $75,000 annually to deploy a Peace Corps volunteer (Campbell, 2004), while a CDC employee costs $250,000–$300,000 per year, including salary (Personal Communication, Michael St. Louis, CDC, February 23, 2005). Moreover, as a large percentage of U.S. health professionals and graduates of higher educational programs graduate with significant debt (Morrison, 2005), the committee believes GHS fellows should be eligible for the GHS Loan Repayment Program (discussed next).

---

[2]The Peace Corps builds diplomacy throughout the world in pursuing its three goals of helping people of interested countries meet their needs for trained men and women, helping to promote a better understanding of Americans on the part of the peoples served, and helping to promote a better understanding of other peoples on the part of all Americans.

[3]This information was received as sample data drawn from the budgets of JHPIEGO. JHPIEGO budgets are based on USAID and State Department rates.

LOAN REPAYMENT PROGRAM

Educational debts are a major problem for many U.S. health personnel, and are a substantial impediment to doctors—and others who accrue similarly large debts—in pursuing volunteer or low-remuneration opportunities such as service abroad in support of the PEPFAR goals. Loan repayment programs are often used to attract health professionals to practice in areas designated as having a shortage of such personnel. In return for service, loan repayment programs offer a percentage of repayment on qualified educational loans with outstanding balances. Federal programs follow guidelines set forth by the Office of Personnel Management, but each agency has specific requirements for service and repayment. Some of the more common loan repayment programs include the NHSC, the U.S. Army Medical Department, and HRSA's Nursing Education Program. Many states also offer loan repayment programs in exchange for service in areas of need (OPM, 2005b). Student loan payments are usually paid directly to the lender, but the payment is included in the employee's gross income and wages for federal employment tax purposes.

Recommendation 6: *Establish a U.S. Global Health Service Loan Repayment Program.* The committee recommends the establishment of a U.S. Global Health Service Loan Repayment Program for clinical, managerial, and technical professionals prepared to serve for designated periods in PEPFAR focus countries. This program would provide $25,000 toward scholastic debt reduction for each year of service in PEPFAR focus countries. Clinical, managerial, and technical professionals graduate from training programs today with substantial debts that limit their ability to consider voluntary or less remunerative work. A loan repayment program would expand the pool of professionals who could consider service abroad and make many more skilled individuals available to address PEPFAR goals.

Program Description

Participants in any of the other GHS programs would be eligible to apply for loan repayment of up to $25,000 per year of service in the PEPFAR focus countries. Service of less than 1 year would not qualify for loan repayment. The implementing or contracted agency of the GHS would manage the Loan Repayment Program and would select recipients on the basis of such criteria as absence of judgment liens arising from federal debt; full-time service (40 hours/week); minimum of a 1-year service period; and if applicable, valid licensure for the country of service.

As is the case under the NHSC loan repayment program, eligible loans could be either federal or commercial, but would have to have been used for educational purposes leading to a relevant degree. If an applicant had a PLUS loan[4] for his or her child, the applicant would be eligible for loan repayment. However, if a PLUS loan were held by an applicant's parent, the applicant would not be eligible for repayment of that loan (OPM, 2005b). Including PLUS loans might encourage midcareer in addition to early-career professionals. A participant who failed to meet the minimum 1-year full-time service requirement would be obligated to repay an amount equal to the sum of the amounts paid by the GHS.

In addition, applicants would have to document that their host organization is a nonprofit entity and that their specific project or initiative contributes to the PEPFAR goals. As with the NHSC loan repayment program, GHS repayments would be exempt from gross income and employment taxes and would not be included as wages in determining benefits under the Social Security Act (NHSC, 2004). Like the Felowship Program, the Loan Repayment Program, would start with 100 awards (roughly 5–10 per PEPFAR focus country, prorated by need) in the first year, but scale up quickly to 1,000 awards by the third year of the program.

Rationale and Evidence

Why a Loan Repayment Program?

In the academic year 1996–1997, medical students borrowed more than $1.11 billion, and 83.2 percent of the 1997 graduating class had educational debt (Beran, 1998). In 2003–2004, tuition and fees at public medical schools averaged $16,153 and at private schools reached a staggering $32,588 (Jolly, 2004). This financial burden could potentially leave a young medical professional with a debt ranging from $140,000 to $255,000, making the concept of exchanging debt for service very appealing (Morrison, 2005).

The NHSC offers professionals an opportunity to compete for repayment of qualified educational loans (see above). In addition to loan repayment, professionals receive a competitive salary and an opportunity to make a difference in an underserved area. Maximum loan repayment during the required 2-year contract is $25,000 per year; participants are eligible to extend loan repayment 1 year at a time based on continued service

---

[4]Parent Loans to Undergraduate Students (PLUS) are loans to parents in order to pay the educational expenses of their child who is a dependent, undergraduate student enrolled at least half time. SOURCE: http://studentaid.ed.gov/.

at a maximum of $35,000 per year for their third year of service and beyond. Payments are made directly to the lender. Clinicians choose their service site before applying to the program, and employment at a site does not guarantee participation in the program. A participant who fails to meet the minimum 2-year full-time service requirement is obligated to pay an amount equal to the sum of the amounts paid by the NHSC for any period of obligated service not served, an amount equal to the number of months of obligated service not completed multiplied by $7,500, and interest on the above amounts at the maximum legal rate (NHSC, 2005).

Similar to the NHSC loan repayment program, the HRSA Nursing Education Loan Repayment Program offers assistance to registered nurses to repay educational loans in exchange for service in facilities with critical shortages. The purpose of this program is to assist in recruiting and retaining professional nurses to work in underserved areas. Applicants must meet strict eligibility requirements, including but not limited to registered nurse (R.N.) status, possession of one or more outstanding loans related to a completed nursing education program, full-time employment in a critical shortage area, possession of a current and unrestricted license to practice in their state of service, U.S. citizenship, absence of any judgment liens, no default on a federal debt, no work for a nurse staffing agency or traveling nurse agency, and no work as faculty at an educational institution. All participants in the loan repayment program must agree to work full time for 2 years in an approved critical-shortage facility. For 2 years of service, 60 percent of the participant's total qualifying loan balance is paid. If a participant completes 2 years of service and decides to work a third year at a critical-shortage facility, the program pays an additional 25 percent of the qualifying loan balance. In contrast to the NHSC approach, payments are made to the participant, who is then responsible for making payments to the lender. The loan repayment program may periodically contact the lender to ensure that payments are being made. Participants who are unable to complete a contract are required to repay all payments made by the program, plus interest at the maximum legal rate (HRSA, 2005; HRSA Bureau of Health Professions, 2005).

Loan repayment is a motivating factor for recruiting and retaining highly skilled professionals to serve in areas of need. Another option, albeit less attractive, is loan deferment or forbearance. Several federal loan programs offer deferments in exchange for Peace Corps service. In addition, volunteers with Perkins loans are eligible for a 15 percent cancellation of their loan balance for each year of Peace Corps service (United States Peace Corps, 2005b). This benefit comes from the loan programs, and the Peace Corps does not actively repay loans in exchange for service. Similarly, full-time service as an officer in the Commissioned Corps of the Public Health Service is rewarded with loan deferment benefits.

Costs

At the level of loan repayment awards envisioned, the costs of the program would start at $2.5 million ($25,000 × 100 awards) and grow to $25 million ($25,000 × 1,000) by the third year of the program, representing less than 0.1 percent of the current PEPFAR budget and less than 1 percent of the projected PEPFAR budget, respectively.

TWINNING PROGRAM

Twinning is a potentially useful tool for building human health care resource capacity in resource-limited settings. It can be particularly helpful when a twinning partnership has been established in a country, and the skills of health professionals can be rapidly engaged through this "instant infrastructure" (USAID, 2001). Such rapid mobilization of U.S. health professionals can fill an immediate need for workers, educators, and trainers while at the same time building a long-term relationship through multiple exchanges over the years. Partnerships whose outcomes involve prevention, treatment, and care for HIV/AIDS can be extremely useful in helping to achieve the PEPFAR goals. These relationships can take many forms, including public–private partnerships, as well as arrangements that involve governments, public health agencies, NGOs, hospitals, and universities. Moving skilled personnel from the United States to organizations in the PEPFAR focus countries offers the potential to build human resource capacity. Likewise, moving health professionals from a host country to a U.S. organization for specific forms of training can result in multiplying the host country's health workforce, provided the training received abroad is appropriate and directly applicable.

Recommendation 7: *Promote twinning as a mechanism to mobilize health personnel.* The committee recommends long-term, targeted funding for innovative, institutional partnerships that would mobilize U.S. health personnel to work in PEPFAR countries. Often called "twinning," these bidirectional partnerships (which encompass counterpart organizations ranging from hospitals and universities to nongovernmental organizations and public health agencies) develop institutional capacities and create a sustainable relationship between the partners that extends beyond the life of the defined project. It is a bilateral arrangement that can develop collaboration in many areas but stands to be a particularly helpful instrument to augment teaching, training, and service capacities in combating HIV/AIDS. Twinning should be supported between a variety of U.S. and PEPFAR country-based institutions that are most relevant to meeting PEPFAR targets and harmonizing with PEPFAR country operating plans, especially public-sector

health agencies. Twinning is a mechanism that can move skilled personnel from a sending organization to a host organization to provide support, training, and technical assistance. It provides a ready-made structure in host countries for U.S. health professionals to engage with maximum speed and effectiveness.

Program Description

Twinning partnerships should target institutions and organizations that national authorities in the PEPFAR focus countries deem to be of strategic importance in building human resources for health. A desire to partner with U.S. organizations should be defined through a country's needs assessment (see above). These partnerships could include relationships with ministries of health, central and district-level health agencies, medical facilities, health education and training institutions, academic centers, and faith- and community-based organizations involved in prevention, treatment, and care for HIV/AIDS.

An in-country coordinator similar to those employed by the European Union could facilitate the twinning process (European Commission Directorate General for Enlargement, 2001). The coordinator would serve as a central point for communication, and would work with PEPFAR teams and national partners to determine which key institutions would most benefit from a twinning partnership. Once the decision had been made to partner with a U.S. organization, the request would be submitted to an intermediary or umbrella organization that would handle all aspects of the subgrant process, including application, selection, orientation, and administration. It would be up to the umbrella organization to find appropriate matches for the requesting country. Matching would be accomplished through a competitive process to attract U.S. participants and to ensure that the proper skill set will be matched with the needs of the focus country. An alternative to using an intermediary would be for organizations to select and arrange their own twinning partnerships. To this end, a large database of all qualifying potential partners could be maintained in the Clearinghouse (discussed in the next section). Organizations in a PEPFAR focus country could, with the help of the in-country coordinator, select a partner from this wide range of choices.

Both partners would have to agree upon a work plan and the process for its implementation before initiating the partnership. The umbrella organization could broker this exchange and monitor its status and progression. The work plan should include agreements on the length of exchanges and the duration of the partnership; Table 5-3 lists advantages and disadvantages of short- and long-term exchanges. Exchanges designed to provide

TABLE 5-3 Advantages and Disadvantages of Short- and Long-Term Exchanges

Length of Exchange	Advantages	Disadvantages
Short-term (2 weeks to 3 months)	• Unpaid volunteers—cost-effective • Funding less of an issue • Opportunity to build institutional memory • Attractive to skilled professionals who cannot commit to long-term service	• Possible problems with follow-up and sustained activities between exchanges • Limited impact of brief engagement • Costs associated with high turnover of personnel
Medium- or long-term (6 months to >12 months)	• Adequate time to develop relationships and earn the trust of key stakeholders • U.S. professionals better equipped to understand and respect the local value system • Facilitates challenging mindsets, vested interests, and power differentials • Opportunity to build institutional capacity	• Lack of funding • Lack of volunteers for long-term stays • Need for substantial compensation for long-term personnel

specific educational instruction could be relatively brief, perhaps lasting 2–3 weeks, whereas those focused on institutional capacity or systems development would likely take longer, at least a year.

All of the exchanges would need to be monitored and evaluated regularly to ensure that both parties are satisfied with the relationship and its results. Evaluations should be conducted by the intermediary organization and might include, for example, measuring the effectiveness of the twinning process, gauging the partnerships' ability to achieve the agreed-upon outcomes, and determining the impact of the partnership on targeted indicators of capacity development (such as the number of health personnel trained to monitor resistance to ART). Evaluations should also address sustainability, which will be essential to the success of any partnership. If a U.S. professional provides training on a specific topic, it is essential to provide follow-up and support to ensure that the participants in the training are able to use their newly acquired skills. This follow-up could be accomplished through either in-country or virtual, online mentoring and support.

Both new and existing partnerships aimed at achieving the PEPFAR goals should be encouraged although new work plans may be needed to reflect such initiatives. Strategies that emphasize targeted and results-driven efforts and can build a foundation for a sustainable relationship should be given the highest priority.

Rationale and Evidence

As noted above, established overseas twinning partnerships offer the advantage of a preexisting infrastructure prepared to receive partners. This ready-made structure can strengthen the host country workforce by allowing the rapid deployment of foreign health professionals to fill personnel voids, to provide relevant side-by-side training with colleagues in their home environment, and to train trainers who can facilitate the dissemination of knowledge in specific areas such as HIV/AIDS prevention and care (ICAD and CI, 2002). The ability to quickly mobilize U.S. personnel can also be used to send relief staff from the United States to substitute temporarily for regular in-country staff while they travel off-site for much needed training. Moreover, twinning can facilitate the development of skills and leadership ability through in-service training and care provision, as well as through on-site or online teaching, coaching, and mentoring.

To facilitate the mobilization of shorter-term professionals, some twinning partners place a key staff member in the host country for at least 12 consecutive months (European Commission Directorate General for Enlargement, 2004). Doing so is particularly helpful in settings in which the health infrastructure is stretched very thin, and no one is available to organize the visiting partner's experience or make logistical arrangements, such as housing. Indeed, relying on the host country partner to do this planning diverts much-needed resources from the provision of health services. Indiana University School of Medicine recognizes this risk and has maintained one full-time clinician at its partner organization, Moi University in Kenya, since 1990 (Einterz et al., 1995). This model has been found to maximum the effectivenees of the partnership by providing continuity and coordination for the large number of shorter-term exchanges that are undertaken, lasting anywhere from weeks to months.

As discussed above, bringing in-country health professionals to a U.S. organization for specific forms of training can multiply the health workforce of the host country. For more than 2 and a half years, for example, New York University (NYU) School of Medicine has been working with organizations in Mombasa and other areas of Kenya to bring physicians to NYU/ Bellevue Hospital Center for leadership and other forms of training focused on HIV/AIDS treatment (Valentine, 2004).

Often, similarly structured groups partner because of the innate learning opportunities; however, groups with organizational differences that share a common goal can also have a successful partnership. An example is the Vietnam–CDC–Harvard Medical School AIDS Partnership. U.S. partners include the CDC Global AIDS Program and the Department of Social Medicine at Harvard Medical School, while activities in Vietnam are coordinated by the AIDS Division of the Ministry of Health and managed through the National Institute for Clinical Research in Tropical Medicine. Although the partners are dissimilar, they have produced positive results and have maintained a long-term relationship (Krakauer, 2004).

The support of public-sector health agencies contributes to the success of HIV/AIDS programs, whether they are orientated toward prevention, treatment, or care. Partnerships may include government entities such as state or local health authorities and public health departments, or organizations of government officials, such as state, district, or provincial AIDS officials, health policy makers, and public managers (World Bank, 2003). Such involvement not only increases the capacity of the local government infrastructure to respond to and manage HIV/AIDS-related activities and the mainstreaming of HIV/AIDS into all aspects of services, but also have the potential to increase the workforce by strengthening leadership and commitment. The Global AIDS Technical Assistance Program of the National Alliance of State and Territorial AIDS Directors, for example, partners its experienced members with country ministries of health and national AIDS control programs, and has thereby gained valuable experience in deploying volunteers and partnering at the governmental level. Since 2000, nearly 50 individuals from 29 U.S. states have provided technical assistance abroad under this program, and nearly one-third of the 50 states have hosted international delegations (NASTAD, 2005).

As noted, twinning relationships such as those described above can be arranged by the organizations themselves or through an intermediary, umbrella organization. Although more expensive, an umbrella organization can have certain advantages over direct funding of partners (see Table 5-4), including having more experience on which to draw. The American International Health Alliance (AIHA), for example, has been the intermediary for partnerships between the United States and Eastern Europe since the end of the cold war in 1992. Through the accumulated experience from its 105 partnerships, AIHA has enlisted more than 5,000 U.S. volunteers to provide 180,000 days of volunteering (Smith, 2005).

Costs

A typical partnership managed through an umbrella organization costs from $200,000 to $350,000 per year, with 65–70 percent of this amount being spent on travel-related expenses (Personal communication, James Smith, AIHA, December 16, 2004). Most of the administrative responsibili-

TABLE 5-4 Advantages and Disadvantages of Partnership Management Models

Model	Advantages	Disadvantages
Umbrella Organization	• Provides a larger pool of special expertise and experience • Has the ability to share knowledge, tools, and lessons learned across partnerships • Permits distillation of procedural requirements • Facilitates grant management • Reduces donor management workload • Donor retains substantive oversight, while management burden is minimized • Promotes equity among partners as not one partner is receiving funds	• Policy priorities may differ (intermediary may press for its own agenda) • Overall costs are higher because of overhead charges • Local or U.S. groups may be reluctant to work through an intermediary • Can create confusion as to roles and functions • Conflict with the intermediary may arise
Direct Partnership	• Provides an opportunity for the donor to shape and guide the emerging relationship • Allows substantive donor involvement in program design and implementation • Permits close monitoring and oversight • More likely to reflect an emphasis consistent with the host country's action plan • Reduces administrative overhead costs	• Heavy management workload • Staff may lack skills or time to nurture partnerships • Host country partner becomes more dependent on the U.S. partner

SOURCE: USAID (2001:13).

ties are on the U.S. side, and as a result, 15–20 percent of the budget often covers the cost of a coordinator who is responsible for reports, work plans, and the like. Host countries do not receive funds for project-related administrative charges they may incur. However, they are often offered learning resource centers that may include information technologies (e.g., computers, Internet connectivity), virtual libraries (e.g., journal subscriptions), and computer and related skills training. For independent partnerships not overseen by an intermediary organization, the required start-up funding is about $350,000. This core funding allows the U.S. partner to pursue the additional funding needed to conduct the twinning project (Einterz, 2004). HRSA has contracted with AIHA to establish twinning partnerships in the PEPFAR focus countries. AIHA plans to develop up to 100 partnerships between the United States and focus countries and up to 50 south-to-south partnerships within the next 5 years (Personal communication, Eun-Joo Chang, AIHA, March 1, 2005).

Benefits

The benefits of twinning extend well beyond the assistance provided to the receiving organization. For the United States, participation in balanced relationships with developing countries serves as a form of public health diplomacy and promotes a positive image of American citizens around the world. Twinning also promotes organizational understanding and cooperation that might otherwise not occur (ICAD and Health Canada, 1999; NASTAD, 2004). On an individual level, participating U.S. health professionals benefit from the opportunity to use their skills in challenging and innovative ways; they also develop skills needed to work in different cultures, as well as in resource-constrained settings (NASTAD, 2004). Moreover, they often gain greater sensitivity to and understanding of immigration and refugee issues in the United States and among their patients. Health professionals participating in twinning programs are in a position to share their experiences with various audiences, raising awareness of HIV/AIDS around the world and at home. Finally, returning health professionals bring with them new perspectives and guidance for their own HIV/AIDS programs, which could translate into improved HIV/AIDS care in the United States (NASTAD, 2004).

Effective relationships established under twinning partnerships can persist over time and remain active despite the coming and going of donors. Such a relationship can grow as it adapts to changes in the environment of both partners. Trust and friendship are underlying factors that make projects successful regardless of the area being addressed.

CLEARINGHOUSE

Many organizations currently send health professionals to work in the PEPFAR focus countries. Given their experience, these groups are well positioned to assist in HIV/AIDS prevention, treatment, and care, thus helping to achieve the PEPFAR goals. The Global Health Service Clearinghouse is designed to assist this community of organizations in mobilizing health personnel to go abroad for HIV/AIDS work. The nature of the HIV/AIDS pandemic has led many organizations that have not previously viewed themselves as "health organizations" to assume a strategic and essential role in testing, counseling, access to treatment, care giving, and the nurture of orphans. The devastation brought about by HIV/AIDS to date and the growing social crisis in many of the PEPFAR focus countries calls for a heightened level of cooperation among individuals and organizations battling the pandemic. Marshaling information technology is crucial to these efforts. The Clearinghouse would help meet this need.

A virtual network of international sending organizations could offer and receive information and regularly reach thousands of volunteers. It woud be an efficient way to use emerging technology to network people and organizations for the benefit of both. For programs located in various and sometimes remote areas, the Clearinghouse would provide a mechanism for recruitment, information posting, and establishment of a global presence. Networking would also enable organizations to share experiences and to work together on common initiatives while minimizing duplication of services.

> Recommendation 8: *Develop a U.S. Global Health Service Clearinghouse.* There are many organizations currently mobilizing health personnel to work in PEPFAR countries. These organizations could be powerful allies in meeting PEPFAR goals. Therefore the committee recommends a multifaceted Clearinghouse for the U.S. Global Health Service that would facilitate information exchange, enhance access to program data, and provide opportunity information for interested health professionals.

Program Description

The Global Health Service Clearinghouse would be managed by a small professional staff working closely with all of the other programs of the GHS. This team would be responsible for developing the virtual and actual networks that would make up the Clearinghouse. Important aspects of the work would include developing and maintaining an inventory of U.S. organizations that mobilize health personnel for deployment in the PEPFAR focus countries, as well as liaising with those performing the health workforce needs assessments discussed earlier. This database would be available to host country counterparts. A more detailed explanation of the four components of the Clearinghouse is presented below.

Program Resource Directory and Networks

As part of an overall website, the Program Resource Directory would be a searchable, web-based directory providing volunteers with screened, reliable links to sending organizations' websites so as to facilitate organizational contacts for recruitment. This function would be especially useful to those applying for a GHS Fellowship or for the Loan Repayment Program, since their applications would be judged in part on their involvement in the program of an established mobilizing organization. Organizations posting links in the Program Resource Directory would be invited to join the network of sending organizations. Being a member would entitle them to participate in a variety of virtual and actual programs, including an annual meeting, an e-newsletter, a Listserv, and other electronic community activities. Organizations involved in twinning partnerships could potentially utilize the networking capabilities established through the Clearinghouse to keep in touch with their sister organization. Groups wishing to be included in this voluntary coordination and communication system of organizations engaged in mobilizing health personnel for the PEPFAR focus counties could self-nominate for inclusion, provided they met basic requirements pertinent to the PEPFAR goals. Criteria for being listed in the directory would be made clear to all organizations.

Opportunity Bank

A job bank of available host country positions would be a vital tool for identifying vacancies that could be filled by U.S. professionals wishing to work in the PEPFAR focus countries. The data in the Opportunity Bank would come from the health workforce needs assessment performed for each focus country (see above). Uniformity of the assessment data will ensure that information sent from the various focus countries will be compatible and comparable for receiving and posting vacancies. Continuous updating of the information posted will be crucial for tracking open positions. The Opportunity Bank offers the potential to serve as a major facilitator of mobilization by both governmental and nongovernmental programs. Its value, however, would depend to a large extent on the quality of the in-country health workforce needs assessment activity and of the link between host country personnel and the Clearinghouse team.

Cultural and Strategic Issues Reference Site

The Cultural and Strategic Issues Reference Site would be a virtual warehouse of information pertinent to all health professionals planning to work in the PEPFAR focus countries, including those seeking a GHS Fellowship, loan repayment, or assignment to the Global Health Service Corps. The site would provide primary information on cultural, political, economic, and social issues for all 15 countries. It would offer a range of relevant documents, including the country strategic plans, country profiles from the Office of the U.S. Global AIDS Coordinator, and related epidemiologic and regional documents for the orientation and edification of potential volunteers.

Crucial information on ethical considerations related to practice abroad would also be provided. A Code for Volunteer Behavior and Conduct could be developed and posted for GHS members to read and sign prior to leaving the United States for work abroad. Statements of policy regarding involvement in local politics and social advocacy activities for GHS-supported personnel might be provided as well.

Country Credentials and Travel Guidelines Repository

Providing potential recruits with credentialing and travel information for work overseas would simplify an often laborious process. The Country Credentials and Travel Guidelines Repository would assist prospective volunteers for work in the global arena by making this information readily available in one virtual location. This regularly updated compendium of information might include country-specific documents regarding licensure, accreditation, and work permits, as well as other helpful information, such as passport, visa, and driver's license requirements; travel information and alerts; and details on travel medical insurance policies.

Rationale and Evidence

The principal rationale for the GHS Clearinghouse is to increase the actual and virtual connectivity of organizations engaged in mobilizing health personnel for service in the PEPFAR focus countries. Many groups in this field have organizational missions and Internet presences that involve promulgating information on volunteer opportunities or country conditions along the lines envisioned for the Clearinghouse. Their activites include the programs of governmental organizations, NGOs, and religious and sectarian organizations listed in Table 5-5.

In analyzing the organizations currently engaging in networking with regard to opportunities for health professionals abroad, it became evident to the committee that no single organization or network addresses all aspects of a comprehensive clearinghouse as described above. Moreover, even similar organizations, such as those linked to religious bodies, rarely focus on the networking and sharing of assets in the recruitment and deployment of health professionals needed to build HIV/AIDS human resource capacity in the PEPFAR focus countries. While the multiple origins and sources of support for these critical organizations explain this relative lack of coordination, the committee believes it important to promote harmonized mobilization efforts where possible and the partnering of organizations when appropriate. The committee believes that the sharing of information envi-

TABLE 5-5 A Sampling of Organizations Providing Information about HIV/AIDS Work Abroad

Organization	Activity
Virtual Matchmaking	
Volunteers for Prosperity http://www.volunteersforprosperity.gov/	Potential volunteers can obtain links to organizations that work in the areas of HIV/AIDS, capacity building, and education.
International Healthcare Opportunities Clearinghouse http://library.umassmed.edu/ihoc/	Provides a web-based database of available positions for health care professionals that is searchable by region, time commitment, language requirement, and professional skills.
International Medical Volunteers Association http://www.imva.org/Pages/volsrchintro.asp	Lists health care opportunities and whom to contact for more information. Provides a volunteer registry that contains information about health professionals seeking volunteer medical assignments around the world.
Networking	
InterAction http://www.interaction.org	A network of more than 160 nongovernmental organizations (NGOs) that convenes and coordinates to affect public policy and improve the outcomes of their work worldwide. They maintain close ties with NGOs and NGO networks in Europe, Asia, Africa, and Latin America.
Uganda Network of AIDS Service Organizations http://www.unaso.or.ug/about.php	A nationwide network of NGOs, community-based organizations, faith-based organizations, groups of people living with HIV/AIDS, and local communities involved in the response to HIV/AIDS in Uganda.
Kenya AIDS NGOs Consortium http://www.kanco.org/framebody.htm	A national membership network of NGOs/community-based organizations and religious organizations involved or with interest in activities related HIV/AIDS and other sexually transmitted infections in Kenya.

TABLE 5-5 Continued

Organization	Activity
Africa Religious Health Assets Program	A collaboration among the University of Cape Town, University of Kwazulu Natal, and Emory University to fill the gap in strategic mapping of religious structures and networks relevant to HIV/AIDS and other underlying health issues.
African Regional Capacity Building Network for HIV/AIDS Prevention, Care, and Treatment (World Bank Group, 2004)	A network of subregional "learning sites" designed to expand training of health care practitioners in HIV/AIDS, and to enable harmonization of approaches and facilitate greater knowledge sharing across Ethiopia, Kenya, and Tanzania.

Virtual Warehousing	
InterAction http://www.interaction.org	Publishes a newsletter; maintains a website with a virtual library, an events calendar listing meetings and locations, and Private Voluntary Organization Standards.
Health Volunteers Overseas http://www.hvousa.org/	Website addresses aspects of volunteering.
Peace Corps http://www.peacecorps.gov/	Website addresses aspects of volunteering.
International Federation of Red Cross and Red Crescent Societies http://www.ifrc.org/what/health/hivaids/code/	Website with a code of good practice for NGOs responding to HIV/AIDS.
U.S. Department of State http://www.state.gov/travel/	Provides extensive information on traveling and living aboard, along with country background notes and key contacts at U.S. embassies and consulates.
Fogarty International http://www.fic.nih.gov/services.html	Provides links to passport and visa information, foreign travel information, and personal security training, as well as available grants.
Development Experience Clearinghouse http://www.dec.org/about.cfm#1	An interactive website of thousands of publications funded by the U.S. Agency for International Development.

continued

TABLE 5-5 Continued

Organization	Activity
International Healthcare Opportunities Clearinghouse http://library.umassmed.edu/ihoc/	Provides links that offer would-be volunteers travel information, as well as information on health and safety risks and history, culture, and customs.
International Clearinghouse on Curriculum for HIV/AIDS Preventive Education http://databases.unesco.org/IBE/AIDBIB/	A bibliographic database of nternational curriculum materials and irelated documentation for HIV/AIDS education at primary and secondary levels of schooling.

sioned for the Clearinghouse would help in maintaining a focus on mobilization goals, preventing duplication of services, and placing volunteers in areas where they would have maximal impact.

As noted, many organizations use websites to provide information about volunteering and working overseas; these sites also allow e-mail communication with the organization and with others in the field. Some sites include databases for use by potential volunteers in matching their skills with the needs of organizations recruiting in various countries. Others display links to websites that offer positions for professional and nonprofessional volunteers (e.g., Volunteers for Prosperity). Some allow volunteers to search based on their specific skill set (e.g., International Healthcare Opportunities Clearinghouse), while others supply the name of a person in the organization for the individual to contact (e.g., International Medical Volunteers Association). Many include opportunities in some PEPFAR focus countries, while Volunteers for Prosperity provides a searchable database of all the PEPFAR focus countries. The website of the International Federation of Red Cross and Red Crescent Societies posts a code of ethics. The website of Fogarty International Center of the National Institutes of Health provides links to passport and visa information, foreign travel information, and personal security information, as does the website of the U.S. Department of State. However, none of these organizations lists both comprehensive information on mobilizing organizations (the proposed Resource Directory) and extensive placement possibilities in the PEPFAR focus countries (the proposed Opportunities Bank). These two features, as well as the ethical, cultural, credentialing, and travel information that would be offered at the GHS Clearinghouse, would bring a coherence not currently available to the complex issues that surround the mobilization of health professionals.

For ease of searching, all four elements of the Clearinghouse should be housed at one website, where those interested could go to be introduced to the various programs of the GHS. The Program Resource Directory and Networks is a likely starting point for sending organizations to become involved with the GHS, and would benefit from a well-designed format such as that of Volunteers for Prosperity or the International Healthcare Opportunities Clearinghouse.

CONCLUDING REMARKS

There have been few well-conducted studies addressing gaps in human resources for health that could guide the U.S. Department of State in determining how many specialized health, management, and technical professionals will be needed to meet the PEPFAR goals. Collecting this information systematically and storing it in a well-maintained database would provide not only a source of information for job vacancies, but also baseline and follow-up data for tracking how well countries are meeting their human resource requirements and thus how well the PEPFAR initiative is meeting its goals. Opportunities for serving in any of the programs of the GHS could also be stored in the virtual database and made available to interested and qualified professionals.

The Global Health Service Corps is likely to be the most expensive of the proposed GHS programs, but is also, the committee believes, the one most likely to have the greatest impact on human resources. The Fellowship and Loan Repayment programs are also expected to increase worker capacity on the ground, as is the Twinning Program, with its unique ability to insert workers into areas or institutions where a partnership has already been developed. Although each program could be implemented independently of the others, the committee believes the greatest impact would come from implementing them collectively, to varying degrees, based on the identified needs of each of the 15 PEPFAR focus countries.

REFERENCES

Adano U, O'Neil M, Decima E, Kiarie W. 2004. *Rapid Assessment of the Human Resource Implications of Scaling up HIV/AIDS Services in Uganda Progress Report 1 & 2.* Management and Leadership Development Project/USAID. Boston, MA: Management Sciences for Health.

Beran RL, Lawson GE. 1998. Medical student financial assistance, 1996–1997. *Journal of the American Medical Association* 280: 819–820.

Campbell R. 2004 (December 2). *Peace Corps.* Presentation at the Institute of Medicine Workshop on Options for Overseas Placement of U.S. Health Professionals, Washington, DC. Institute of Medicine Committee on the Options for Overseas Placement of U.S. Health Professionals.

CDC (Centers for Disease Control and Prevention). 2005. *Global AIDS Program Country and Regional Programs*. [Online]. Available: http://www.cdc.gov/nchstp/od/gap/ countries/ [accessed March 10, 2005].

CIES (Council for International Exchange of Scholars). 2005. *The Fulbright Program*. [Online]. Available: http://www.cies.org/about_fulb.htm [accessed February 22, 2005].

Diallo K, Zurn P, Gupta N, Dal Poz M. 2003. Monitoring and evaluation of human resources for health: An international perspective. *Human Resources for Health* 1(3).

Einterz R. 2004 (December 2). *Partnering: University to University Training*. Presentation at the Institute of Medicine Workshop on the Options for the Overseas Placement of U.S. Health Professionals, Washington, DC. Institute of Medicine Committee on the Overseas Placement of U.S. Health Professionals.

Einterz RM, Kelley CR, Mamlin JJ, Van Reken DE. 1995. Partnerships in international health: The Indiana University–Moi University experience. *Infectious Disease Clinics of North America* 9(2):453–455.

European Commission Directorate General for Enlargement. 2001. *Twinning in Action*. Brussels, Belgium: European Commission Directorate General for Enlargement.

European Commission Directorate General for Enlargement. 2004. *Institution Building in the Framework of European Union Policies: A Reference Manual on 'Twinning' Projects*. European Union: European Commission Directorate General for Enlargement.

FHI (Family Health International). 2003. *Baseline Assessment Tools for Preventing Mother-to-Child Transmission of HIV*. Research Triangle Park, NC: FHI.

Fogarty International Center. 2002 (October 31). *AIDS International Training and Research Program Announcement PA-03-018*. [Online]. Available: http://grants2.nih.gov/grants/ guide/pa-files/PA-03-018.html [accessed February 22, 2005].

HLF (High Level Forum on the Health Millennium Development Goals). 2004. *Health Workforce Challenges: Lessons from Country Experiences*. Abuja, Nigeria: World Bank and WHO.

HRSA (Health Resources and Administration). 2005. *Nursing Education Loan Repayment Program Fiscal Year 2005 Application Kit*. [Online]. Available: ftp://ftp.hrsa.gov/bhpr/ nelrp/nelrpapplication05.pdf [accessed February 17, 2005].

HRSA Bureau of Health Professions. 2005. *Nursing Education Loan Repayment Program*. [Online]. Available: http://bhpr.hrsa.gov/nursing/loanrepay.htm [accessed February 17, 2005].

Huddart J, Furth R, Lyons JV. 2004. *The Zambia HIV/AIDS Workforce Study: Preparing for Scale-Up*. Operations Research Results. Bethesda, MD: Quality Assurance Project, University Research Co., LLC.

ICAD and CI (Inter-agency Coalition on AIDS and Development and Communication Initiative). 2002. *Twinning Against AIDS*. Quebec, Canada: Canadian International Development Agency. [Online]. Available: http://www.comminit.com/pdf/twinning_against_ AIDS_Final_Report.pdf [accessed March 11, 2005].

ICAD and Health Canada. 1999. *Beyond Our Borders: A Guide to Twinning for HIV/AIDS Organizations*. Ottowa, Ontario: Interagency Coalition on AIDS and Development. [Online]. Available: http://www.icad-cisd.com/pdf/twinning.pdf [accessed March 11, 2005].

IHS (Indian Health Service). 2005. *Indian Health Service*. [Online]. Available: http://www. ihs.gov/ [accessed March 17, 2005].

IMVA (International Medical Volunteers Association). 2005. *The IMVA Volunteer Registry*. [Online]. Available: http://imva.org/pages/volsrchintro.asp [accessed March 10, 2005].

Interim Pharmacy Council of South Africa. 1998. *The Production and Distribution of Human Resources in Pharmacy*. Durban, South Africa: Health Systems Trust.

IOM (Institute of Medicine). 2005. *Scaling Up Treatment for the Global AIDS Pandemic.* Washington, DC: The National Academies Press.

Jolly P. 2004. *Medical School Tuition and Young Physician Indebtedness.* Washington, DC: AAMC.

Katerere D, Matowe L. 2003. Effect of pharmacist emigration on pharmaceutical services in southern Africa. *American Journal of Health-System Pharmacy* 60:1169–1170.

Kelly N. 2004 (December 2). *Health Volunteers Overseas.* Presentation at the Institute of Medicine Workshop on the Options for the Overseas Placement of U.S. Health Professionals, Washington, DC. Institute of Medicine Committee on the Overseas Placement of U.S. Health Professionals.

Kober K, Van Damme W. 2004. Scaling up access to antiretroviral treatment in southern Africa: Who will do the job? *Lancet* 364:103–107.

Kombe G, Galaty D, Nwagbara C. 2004. *Scaling Up Antiretroviral Treatment in the Public Sector in Nigeria: A Comprehensive Analysis of Resource Requirements.* Bethesda, MD: The Partners for Health Reform Plus Project, Abt. Associates, Inc.

Krakauer E. 2004 (December 2). *Human Resource Needs for HIV Treatment in Vietnam.* Presentation at the Institute of Medicine Workshop on the Options for the Overseas Placement of U.S. Health Professionals, Washington, DC. Institute of Medicine Committee on the Overseas Placement of U.S. Health Professionals.

Morrison G. 2005. Mortgaging our future: The cost of medical education. *New England Journal of Medicine* 352(2):117–119.

MSH (Management Sciences for Health). 1998. *Human Resource Development (HRD) Assessment Instrument for Non-Governmental Organizations (NGOs) and Public Sector Health Organizations.* Boston, MA: Management Sciences for Health.

MSH. 2003. *Human Resource Management Rapid Assessment Tool for HIV/AIDS Environments: A Guide for Strengthening HRM Systems.* Boston, MA: Management Sciences for Health.

MSH. 2004. Tackling the crisis in human capacity development for health services. *Manager* 13(2):1–20.

NASTAD (National Alliance of State and Territorial AIDS Directors). 2004. *International Twinning and Technical Assistance Projects: How Do U.S. State HIV/AIDS Programs Benefit?* [Online]. Available: http://www.nastad.org/documents/public/HIVInternational Programs/200497nternationalTwinningandTechnicalAssistance Projects.pdf [accessed February 28, 2005].

NASTAD. 2005. *NASTAD Global AIDS TA Program: Frequently Asked Questions.* [Online]. Available: http://www.nastad.org/documents/public/HIVInternationalPrograms/2005126 GlobalTAFactSheet.pdf [accessed February 28, 2005].

NHSC (National Health Service Corps). 2003. *About NHSC.* [Online]. Available: http:// nhsc.bhpr.hrsa.gov/about/ [accessed March 10, 2005].

NHSC. 2004. *NHSC Loan Repayment Program Frequently Asked Questions FY 2005.* [Online]. Available: ftp://ftp.hrsa.gov/nhsc/faq/FAQ-LRP-05-ver01.pdf#page=1 [accessed February 17, 2005].

NHSC. 2005. *NHSC Loan Repayment Program Fiscal Year 2005 Applicant Information Bulletin.* [Online]. Available: ftp://ftp.hrsa.gov/nhsc/applications/lrp_05/2005LRP Bulletin.pdf [accessed February 17, 2005].

Ntuli A, Ijumba P, McCoy D, Padarath A, Berthiaume L. 2003. *HIV/AIDS and Health Sector Responses in South Africa—Treatment Access and Equity: Balancing the Act.* Durban, South Africa: Health Systems Trust.

OPM (Office of Personnel Management). 2005a. *Salary Table 2005-GS.* [Online]. Available: http://www.opm.gov/oca/05tables/pdf/gs.pdf [accessed March 17, 2005].

OPM. 2005b. *Federal Student Loan Repayment Program.* [Online]. Available: http://
www.opm.gov/oca/PAY/StudentLoan [accessed February 17, 2005].

Palmer B. 2004 (December 2). *Potential Future Volunteers: Issues and Obstacles to Service.*
Presentation at the Institute of Medicine Workshop on the Options for the Overseas
Placement of U.S. Health Professionals, Washington, DC. Institute of Medicine Commit-
tee on the Overseas Placement of U.S. Health Professionals.

PHRplus (Partners for Health Reform Plus). 2004. *Nigeria: Rapid Assessment of HIV/AIDS
Care in the Public and Private Sectors.* Bethesda, MD: The Partners for Health Reform
Plus Project, Abt. Associates, Inc.

RATN. 2003. *Eastern and Southern Africa Regional HIV/AIDS Training Needs Assessment
Regional Report.* [Online]. Available: http://www.ratn.org/reports/Regional%20
Report.pdf [accessed March 1, 2005].

Rieffel L. 2003. *The Peace Corps in a Turbulent World: A Working Paper.* Washington, DC:
Brookings Institution.

Smith J. 2005 (February 14). *Working in a PEPFAR Context.* Presentation at the Institute of
Medicine Workshop on the Options for the Overseas Placement of U.S. Health Professionals, Washington, DC. Institute of Medicine Committee on the Overseas Placement
of U.S. Health Professionals.

South Africa Ministry of Health. 2003. *Operational Plan for Comprehensive HIV and AIDS
Care, Management and Treatment for South Africa.* Pretoria, South Africa: South Africa
Department of Health.

SWEF (Systemwide Effects of the Fund) Research Network. 2005. *Measuring the Effects of
the Global Fund on Broader Health Systems.* Bethesda, MD: PHRplus. [Online]. Available: http://www.phrplus.org/Pubs/SWEF2_fin.pdf [accessed March 18, 2005].

United States Peace Corps. 2005a. *About the Peace Corps.* [Online]. Available: http://www.
peacecorps.gov/index.cfm?shell=learn.whatispc.fastfacts [accessed February 22, 2005].

United States Peace Corps. 2005b. *Financial Benefits and Loan Deferment.* [Online]. Available: http://www.peacecorps.gov/index.cfm?shell=learn.whyvol.finben [accessed February 17, 2005].

USAID (United States Agency for International Development). 2001. *Designing and Managing Partnerships between U.S. and Host-Country Entities.* Arlington, VA: USAID Development Experience Clearinghouse.

USAID. 2003. *The Health Sector Human Resource Crisis in Africa: An Issues Paper.* Washington, DC: Academy for Educational Development SARA Project.

USAID Guyana. 2003. *Country Strategic Plan 2004–2008.* Guyana, South Africa: USAID.
[Online]. Available: http://www.dec.org/pdf_docs/PDACA685.pdf [accessed March 10,
2005].

Valentine F. 2004 (December 2). *Training Kenyan Healthcare Workers: An Academic Per-
spective.* Presentation at the Institute of Medicine Workshop on the Options for the
Overseas Placement of U.S. Health Professionals, Washington, DC. Institute of Medicine
Committee on the Overseas Placement of U.S. Health Professionals.

Vastag B. 2002. Volunteers see the world and help its people. *Journal of the American
Medical Association* 288(5):559–565.

Weaver DR. 2004 (December 2). *National Health Service Corps.* Presentation at the Institute
of Medicine Workshop on the Options for the Overseas Placement of U.S. Health Professionals, Washington, DC. Institute of Medicine Committee on the Overseas Placement of U.S. Health Professionals.

World Bank. 2003. *Local Government Responses to HIV/AIDS: A Handbook.* Washington,
DC: World Bank.

World Bank Group. 2004. *Africa: World Bank Supports Capacity-Building for HIV/AIDS Prevention, Treatment and Care in Ethiopia, Kenya, and Tanzania.* [Online]. Available: http://web.worldbank.org/WBSITE/EXTERNAL/COUNTRIES/AFRICAEXT/ KENYAEXTN/0,,contentMDK:20266665~menuPK:356530~pagePK:141137~piPK: 141127~theSitePK:356509,00.html [accessed April 30, 2005].

WHO (World Health Organization). 2002. *World Health Organization ARV Toolkit.* [Online]. Available: http://www.who.int/hiv/toolkit/arv/en/content.jsp?ID=193& d=arv. 06.01 [accessed March 10, 2005].

WHO. 2003. *World Health Report 2003.* Geneva, Switzerland: WHO. [Online]. Available: http://www.who.int/whr/2003/en/whr03_en.pdf [accessed March 10, 2005].

WHO. 2004. *Scaling Up HIV/AIDS Care: Service Delivery and Human Resources Perspectives.* Geneva, Switzerland: WHO.

Wyss K. 2004a. *Scaling Up Antiretroviral Treatment and Human Resources for Health: What Are the Challenges in sub-Saharan Africa?* Berne, Switzerland: Swiss Agency for Development and Cooperation.

Wyss K. 2004b. *Human Resources for Health Development for Scaling-Up Antiretroviral Treatment in Tanzania.* Basel, Switzerland: Swiss Tropical Institute.

6

Looking Ahead

Sustainable solutions to the human resources crisis in addressing global HIV/AIDS will ultimately come from highly affected countries. The Global Health Service (GHS) and component programs proposed in this report could play an important role in catalyzing solutions to the crisis in the PEPFAR focus countries. At the same time, the committee anticipates that GHS personnel and programs—being country-responsive and mission-driven—would adjust to changing conditions over time as the pandemic recedes, and new indigenous workers and configurations of care emerge on the ground. In other words, although an exit timetable cannot be forecast at this stage of the pandemic, the committee endorses the principle of flexible downsizing over time.

This final chapter discusses a long-term view of capacity development, creative partnerships, value-added investments (e-health and global health education), ethical issues in foreign health workforce assistance, and monitoring and evaluation.

A LONG-TERM VIEW OF CAPACITY DEVELOPMENT

The GHS is envisioned as a strategic and humanitarian intervention in settings that currently lack sufficient human health care resources to mount a counterattack on HIV/AIDS. The six programs of the GHS are not intended to produce a permanent workforce or to substitute for the development of health personnel capacity in the PEPFAR focus countries. The long-term sustainability of the program must be a priority for both the PEPFAR countries and the United States. Over time, all the PEPFAR countries will have to develop sufficiently capable and sustainable workforces to continue HIV/AIDS prevention and treatment programs into the foreseeable future. There is a strong rationale for U.S. health professionals, as well as other foreign workers, to help through training, skill development, partnership, and other forms of human resource support.

The committee believes that national capacity development in each PEPFAR focus country should entail the following steps:

1. Each country should undertake a health workforce needs assessment as part of or a complement to its national plan. National plans are necessary to orient human resource investments and the filling of gaps by foreign personnel. The needs assessment should encompass not only HIV/AIDS, but also primary prevention and care, because indigenous workers need to pursue their career development within a national system and strategy.

2. National education and training should be accelerated to develop the human resources needed to address the HIV/AIDS pandemic and meet primary health care needs. Those personnel likely to be in highest demand are paraprofessionals such as community health workers. U.S. personnel can contribute to this massive training mission through regionally based activities that maximize the use of available trainers. This contribution is particularly important in sparsely populated areas that lack broad and effective educational and training institutions.

3. The work environment for health professionals should ensure staff retention and promote staff performance. To this end, attention must be paid to financial and nonfinancial incentives, especially social recognition for work performed (Vujicic et al., 2004). Note, however, that special payments to national staff should be viewed with caution; while motivating some, they could discourage others.

4. The "brain drain" should be stemmed by the dampening of demand in richer countries that continue to recruit health workers. Two important measures to this end are developing codes of conduct for the recruitment of health professionals and working toward self-sufficiency in the production of health workers (Buchan et al., 2003; Stilwell et al., 2004).

5. Where necessary, priority programs and health systems should be harmonized to avoid fragmentation, duplication, and waste. With more than half of total health expenditures in some PEPFAR focus countries coming from foreign sources, U.S. personnel can enhance harmonization of funders and funding activities through policy and management support.

Although the development of long term-health professional capacity must be a priority for host countries, the United States can take significant actions to assist in the effort. Foremost among these is investing in the develoment of indigenous health workforce capacity. Medical and nursing schools need to be built and staffed. Midlevel provider programs that offer continuing education and advanced training need to be promoted and funded. Community and village health workers need to be trained by the thousands and equipped with standardized basic skills for HIV/AIDS work. Training programs at all levels for special competencies associated with HIV/AIDS care need to be supported. PEPFAR, as well as the programs of other agencies of the U.S. government, U.S. philanthropies, corporations, nongovernmental organizations (NGOs), and private donors, should all focus on this crucial and central mission. The United States should collaborate with other governments and those in the global donor community to plan and coordinate a massive health personnel training campaign for countries highly impacted by HIV/AIDS.

A second way in which the United States could play a key role in creating stability in the health sector of developing countries is by helping to end the brain drain. Developing nations often experience a chronic and sometimes severe loss of physicians, nurses, and other professionals to developed nations. Among other factors, this migration out of the focus countries is triggered by the failure of the United States and other developed nations to educate sufficient health professionals to meet their domestic needs (Stilwell et al., 2004). The developed countries then must rely on foreign-trained physicians and nurses to close their gaps in service. The resultant exodus of scarce human health care resources is a prominent barrier to building clinical cadres in the PEPFAR focus countries to assume the increased demands of HIV/AIDS, prevention, treatment, and care.

In summary, the committee believes that:

• PEPFAR and other governmental and nongovernmental programs in the United States and elsewhere should invest heavily in programs to build health professional capacity in countries highly impacted by HIV/ AIDS. These investments should include the funding of training programs, instructors, faculty development, and construction where necessary.

• The U.S. government should work with other governments and international donor organizations in collaboration with the PEPFAR focus countries to mount a strategic campaign for the training of health personnel.

• The United States and other developed nations should make a formal commitment to self-sufficiency in meeting their health workforce needs and embark promptly on the training programs necessary to meet this commitment.

• Over the short term, the United States and other developed nations should avoid explicit or implicit recruitment strategies that target the health care workers of low-income countries.

CREATIVE PARTNERSHIPS

Increasingly employed in comprehensive development frameworks, public–private partnerships have featured prominently in international health in recent years. In 2003, the database of the Initiative on Public–Private Partnerships for Health of the Global Forum for Health Research listed 91 international arrangements in the health sector that qualified as public–private partnerships; 76 of these were dedicated to the prevention and control of infectious diseases, notably AIDS, tuberculosis, and malaria (Nishtar, 2004). Large partnerships can also be hosted by an NGO, or can be formed between individual governments and the private sector or NGOs with particular technical or outreach strengths.

In principle, as long as one private for-profit organization and at least one not-for-profit organization share efforts and benefits in pursuit of a common objective for the creation of social value, their collaboration can be deemed a public–private partnership. In the United States alone, hundreds of millions of dollars has been invested to promote partnerships creating "thousands of alliances, coalitions, consortia and other health partnerships" (Lasker et al., 2001:179). To support the health workforce mission of PEPFAR, a variety of creative public-private partnerships can be envisioned. One outstanding example currently targeting human capacity gaps with corporate know-how is the Pfizer Global Health Fellows program (described in detail in Chapter 3). Similarly, innovative human resource collaborations are possible with respect to managing laboratory assets, creating reliable drug delivery systems, and redesigning local health care delivery systems. Table 6-1 provides an overview of companies and organizations currently addressing HIV/AIDS in the PEPFAR focus countries. The interventions listed focus on voluntary counseling and testing; prevention, education and awareness; and care, support and treatment. However, these organizations may also be interested in human resource issues and other activities aimed at achieving the PEPFAR goals.

Creating a true partnership requires mutual understanding and reciprocity among all parties entering into the relationship. Thus all parties should have something to offer and something to gain, and should avoid the unspoken assumption that the one with the resources wields the power. It may even be necessary to compensate intentionally for the imbalance of power to promote communication and avoid relationships of dependency and paternalism. Those involved in public–private partnerships need to be especially cognizant of cross-cultural differences regarding schedules, efficiency, and structure.

TABLE 6-1 Potential Partners Addressing HIV/AIDS

Company/Organization	Intervention
Coca-Cola Company http://www2.coca-cola.com/citizenship/ africa_program.html	Voluntary counseling and testing (VCT); prevention, education, and awareness (PEA); care, support, and treatment (CST)
Voxiva http://www.voxiva.net/solutions_hiv_aid.html#desc03	PEA
Merck http://www.merck.com/about/cr/policies_performance/ social/medicines_developing.html	PEA, CST
Levi Strauss http://www.levistrauss.com/responsibility/ foundation/index.htm	PEA, CST
IBM http://www.weforum.org/pdf/Initiatives/GHI_HIV_ CaseStudy_IBM.pdf	VCT, PEA, CST
Abbott Laboratories http://www.abbott.com	VCT, PEA, CST
GlaxoSmithKline http://www.gsk.com/community/index.htm	PEA, CST

SOURCE : Global Business Coalition on HIV/AIDS (2005).

VALUE-ADDED INVESTMENTS

In considering how to further the capacity-building mission in global health, the committee discussed two strategies that did not rise to the level of formal recommendations, but would be important value-added investments.

E-Health

E-health is defined as the use of technology to exchange actionable information to facilitate the delivery of health services (Ladd, 2005). E-health broadly encompasses the following:

• Telemedicine—the use of technology to support the delivery of clinical services (e.g., telesurgery)

- Telehealth—the use of technology to support a wide range of health-related communications and information exchanges (e.g., teleconsultations)
- Information and communications technologies for health—the use of technology to realize time and cost efficiencies in day-to-day practice (e.g., routine data collection using handheld computers)

While this report addresses information management and information technology primarily through the proposed GHS Clearinghouse, the committee also recognizes the great potential for e-health to mitigate the human capacity shortfall by enabling health care workers to increase their efficiency and effectiveness, providing the local health care establishment with immediate access to experts and expert centers in the United States and elsewhere, and offering individual support to deployed professionals to enable and encourage deployments of longer duration. The committee received written and verbal testimony regarding e-health (see Appendixes E and F). Key points regarding the relevance of e-health to the workforce expansion effort are summarized below.

E-health allows health professionals to overcome time and distance barriers, bringing expertise, education, and training to remote locations and providing services that poor, isolated communities would otherwise lack. In December 2004, the World Health Organization endorsed the use of e-health (WHO, 2004). A specific e-health application (among many) that could support the scale-up of HIV/AIDS treatment and care in the PEPFAR focus countries is the use of interactive personal digital assistants (PDAs) for management of antiretroviral therapy (ART), patient record keeping, patient tracking, larger-scale data collection, and knowledge building. A pilot evaluation of this technology is currently under way in remote villages of Uganda, allowing health professionals there to share information and data with colleagues in Kampala.

One of the main challenges in applying e-health strategies to extend workforce capacity in the PEPFAR focus countries will be to suit the technology and hardware to the context in which care is being delivered. As discussed in Appendix E, sources of connectivity for e-health include satellites, local Internet services, landline phone networks, cellular phone networks, broadcast and two-way radios, WiFi and WiMax networks, and "sneaker networks."[1] Hardware components include desktop computers, laptop computers, handheld computers, satellite ground stations, access points, smart phones, pagers/Blackberries, cell phones, satellite phones, and

---

[1] "Sneaker networks" refers to connectivity via motorbike, bicycle, and foot.

landline phones. Consequently, many possible configurations may be proposed. A basic principle underlying all e-health interventions is that they should be collaborative and constructive, resulting in clear benefits rather than increasing the workload of already overwhelmed workers.

Despite the human and technological challenge of designing e-health interventions to complement different workplaces, the committee strongly believes that e-health can leverage health care resources in the PEPFAR focus countries. The committee therefore endorses the testing of potentially replicable e-health models in the scale-up of HIV/AIDS treatment and care.

Global Health Education in the United States

International health is more than the study of diseases of the developing world; it is a matrix of many contributing factors—chief among them economic, cultural, historical, political, and environmental—that also influence health and disease worldwide. Students of international health therefore benefit from a multidisciplinary approach.

Schools of nursing were early innovators in the area of international health, particularly in their focus on transcultural aspects. These concepts and, in some instances, specific graduate specialty programs have been interwoven throughout undergraduate and graduate curricula in most schools. A few nursing schools have joint graduate degree programs with schools of public health in the area of international health.

Current interest in international health among U.S. medical students and postgraduate residents is also running high. More than 20 percent of students graduating from U.S. medical schools in 2003 participated in an international health experience during their undergraduate medical training, compared with just 6 percent of students graduating in 1984 (AAMC, 1984, 2003). In general, students pursue such experiences to fill perceived gaps in their education, to achieve cross-cultural understanding, or to satisfy altruistic ideals (Taylor, 1994).

Today, students are also interested in international health research. In 2004, the first 20 highly competitive participants were selected for a new Fogarty/Ellison Fellowship in Global Health and Clinical Research Training, a 1-year mentored clinical research experience at an established National Institutes of Health–funded research center in a developing country. This program is open to any U.S. medical, osteopathic, public health, nursing, or dentistry student.[2] The Yale/Johnson and Johnson Physician Scholar

---

[2]Fourteen sites that met stringent criteria for research training were selected for the initial fellowship year: Botswana, Brazil, Haiti, India (2), Kenya, Mali, Peru (2), South Africa (2), Thailand, Uganda, and Zambia. Information about Fogarty/Ellison Fellowships is available at: http://www.aamc.org/students/medstudents/overseasfellowship/2004recipients.htm.

Award sends 80 residents and senior physicians abroad on an elective rotation each year. It has been found that overseas experiences during early professional life often lead to career choices in public health and an increased commitment to underserved populations both in the United States and in other countries (Gupta et al., 1999).

These examples and others suggest there could be a sizeable pool of U.S. health professionals seeking overseas work opportunities linked to global service in the future. To better serve their educational and employment needs, upgraded global health curricula, supported by appropriate professional consortia, should be encouraged, within both health professional schools and other educational settings.

In most U.S. colleges and universities, global health electives, courses, and degree programs are situated within medical schools and schools of public health. Unfortunately, these programs have not received the benefit of support from federal health professions legislation (Titles VII and VIII of the United States Public Health Service Act). Because virtually all of the support provided under this legislation has been targeted at developing the U.S.-based workforce to meet the health needs of this country, little or no attention has been paid to the development of international health expertise. With the exception of certain organizations, such as the International Health and Medical Education Consortium (see Box 6-1), there is little connectivity among students, teachers, course directors, and curricula in the area of international health. The information base on global health study programs outside of graduate schools of health is even sparser. Some universities offer interdepartmental majors in international development or global studies. Standardized, multidisciplinary educational offerings combining, for example, anthropology, economics, environmental sciences, management, and political science, would complement programs aimed at long-term U.S. capacity development in several sectors, including health.

As evidence of this growing need, in February 2005 Fogarty International Center invited applications for new programs aimed at fostering global health research and teaching, possibly to include new multidisciplinary global health curricula for undergraduates and graduates in U.S. universities (NIH, 2005). Similar trends overseas have led, for example, to a new bachelor of science degree in global health as one option for completing the bachelor of medicine and bachelor of surgery degree in the United Kingdom (Bateman et al., 2001; Yudkin et al., 2003). The committee supports enhanced investments in such educational offerings and encourages the development of new multidisciplinary curricula in the United States to prepare the next generation of professionals to address HIV/AIDS and other global health challenges likely to arise in the coming decades.

BOX 6-1
International Health and Medical Education Consortium

International Health and Medical Education Consortium (IHMEC), a nonprofit organization, is a consortium of health professionals, faculty, health educators, and institutions dedicated to international health and medical education. Formed in 1991, its mission is to foster medical education in international health in four program areas—curricula, clinical training, career development, and international education policy.

IHMEC members represent 82 medical schools, primarily in the United States and Canada, that participate in four general programs areas: global health education policy, curriculum development, clinical electives locally and abroad, and national and international institutional partnerships. Its more than 500 individual members include students, faculty, and other health professionals, and there is also a mailing list of more than 1,000 physicians, nurses, public health officers, physician assistants, and health educators interested in global health. In addition to medical schools, IHMEC partners with schools of nursing and public health; international health institutions worldwide; and professional associations representing public health practitioners, nurse practitioners, and physician assistants.

Through its focus on education, IMHEC fosters global health leadership by educating, training, and mentoring students, faculty, professionals, and practitioners to address global health challenges.

SOURCES: Stuck et al. (1995) and Velji (1991).

ETHICAL CONSIDERATIONS IN DEPLOYING
U.S. HEALTH PROFESSIONALS OVERSEAS

For many reasons that are discussed throughout this report, addressing the human health care resource crisis in the battle against global HIV/AIDS is a humanitarian and political imperative (see in particular the discussion in Chapter 2). The committee believes that deploying U.S. health professionals to help with training, skill building, and other forms of partnership can greatly contribute to achieving the PEPFAR goals and building primary health care systems in highly affected countries. However, the committee also recognizes the need to consider the ethical aspects of a large-scale deployment of U.S. health professionals. In December 2004, the committee heard testimony on ethical issues involved in foreign health workforce assistance programs (for the full testimony, see Appendix B). This section summarizes key points from this testimony many of which also appear in Chapter 4.

Models of emergency humanitarian intervention vary widely. They range from short-term emergency efforts (during civil disorders, for example, when health systems are nonfunctioning), to small-scale assistance (the current reality in many PEPFAR focus countries), to large-scale comprehensive assistance with overall strategic coordination. The GHS programs proposed in this report fall into the third of these categories, with training as their paramount mission. The central equity-related question arising from this mission is whether U.S. or other volunteer health personnel focused on a vertical HIV/AIDS program will inadvertently fuel brain drain and/or displace local practitioners from other essential work, including primary health care. To address this issue, the committee supports national human resource planning for health that encompasses not only HIV/AIDS, but also primary prevention and care, as discussed earlier in this chapter.

Another relevant equity issue arises from the principle of "primum non nocere" (first do no harm). Without sustainability, short-term assistance could result in even greater disarray in national health systems, as well as feelings of abandonment on the part of host countries.

Other ethical issues facing U.S. health personnel overseas includes setting priorities and selecting beneficiaries (volunteers may have different standards than host countries and counterparts regarding men, women, young children, and stigmatized groups as targets for HIV/AIDS treatment and care). Moreover, motivations (for example, political or religious beliefs) may differ between participating U.S. health personnel and the funders of PEPFAR.

MONITORING AND EVALUATION

The recent rapid increase in international funding to battle the HIV/AIDS pandemic and other major sources of global disease burden, including malaria and tuberculosis, has made monitoring and evaluation capacity essential to ensure that resources are used effectively at the national and subnational levels. Components of monitoring and evaluation capacity for international initiatives addressing international diseases include overall systems, biologic surveillance, behavioral surveillance, research, program monitoring, and financial monitoring.

With respect to the proposed GHS, monitoring and evaluation would clearly be important, and would require flexible systems to assess and track the work of various program participants. These findings, in turn, would guide adjustments in numbers of personnel, professional and personal qualifications, and other skill sets so as to achieve the greatest benefit in augmenting the health workforce in the PEPFAR focus countries.

The committee was not in a position to design precise monitoring and evaluation instruments for each proposed program of the GHS, nor would this be a practical exercise at this stage. However, the committee did reflect upon a provocative question posed by a key PEPFAR official: "What would success on the ground look like?" Apart from the 5-year numeric targets of PEPFAR, the committee believes the following criteria could be considered a reasonable measure of success:

- Satisfaction among PEPFAR recipients and GHS participants, and the productivity of U.S. health personnel
- Skills and knowledge of PEPFAR country counterparts
- Perceptions of host organizations (public- and private-sector)
- Perceptions of general stakeholder communities in the PEPFAR focus countries
- International dissemination of successful models
- New paradigms of care and configurations of service providers for HIV/AIDS prevention, treatment, and care in all countries heavily impacted by the pandemic

With respect to the broader philosophical framework of monitoring and evaluation, two final principles are worth emphasizing. First, to ensure sustainable collaborations, the programs of the GHS must be useful to society, and their value must flow to all core partners. Second, the envisioned partnerships must be viewed as a continual learning process, with the potential for offering unexpected lessons. Strategically strengthening a country's capacity to monitor and evaluate its workforce is a potentially sustainable effort that would be mutually beneficial to all countries.

REFERENCES

AAMC (Association of American Medical Colleges). 1984. *Medical School Graduation Questionnaire All Schools Report*. Washington, DC: AAMC.

AAMC. 2003. *Medical School Graduation Questionnaire All Schools Report*. Washington, DC: AAMC.

Bateman C, Baker T, Hoornenborg E, Ericsson U. 2001. Bringing global issues to medical teaching. *Lancet* 358(9292):1539–1542.

Buchan J, Parkin T, Sochalski J. 2003. *International Nurse Mobility: Trends and Policy Implications*. Geneva, Switzerland: WHO.

Global Business Coalition on HIV/AIDS. 2005. *Global Business Coalition on HIV/AIDS*. [Online]. Available: http://www.businessfightsaids.org/site/pp.asp?c=nmK0LaP6E&b=202243 [accessed March 17, 2005].

Gupta AR, Wells CK, Horwitz RI, Bia FJ, Barry M. 1999. The international health program: The fifteen-year experience with Yale University's Internal Medicine Residency Program. *American Journal of Tropical Medicine & Hygiene* 61(6):1019–1023.

Ladd H. 2005 (February 14). *Telemedicine and Telehealth*. Presentation at the February 14, 2005, Workshop of the IOM Committee on Options for the Overseas Placement of U.S. Health Professionals, Washington, DC.

Lasker RD, Weiss ES, Miller R. 2001. Partnership synergy: A practical framework for studying and strengthening the collaborative advantage. *Milbank Quarterly* 79:179–205.

NIH (National Institute of Health). 2005. *Framework Programs for Global Health.* [Online]. Available: http://grants.nih.gov/grants/guide/pa-files/PAR-05-050.html [accessed March 1, 2005].

Nishtar S. 2004. Public–private "partnerships" in health: A global call to action. *Health Research Policy and Systems* 2:5. [Online]. Available: http:www.health-policy-systems. com/contents/2/1/5 [accessed March 1, 2005].

Stilwell B, Diallo K, Zurn P, Vujicic M, Adams O, Dal Poz M. 2004. Migration of health care workers from developing countries: Strategic approaches to its management. *Bulletin of the World Health Organization* 82(8).

Stuck C, Bickley L, Wallace N, Velji AM. 1995. International Health Medical Education Consortium: Its history, philosophy, and role in medical education and health development. *Infectious Disease Clinics of North America* 9(3):419–423.

Taylor CE. 1994. International experience and idealism in medical education. *Academic Medicine* 69(8):631–634.

Velji AM. 1991. International health beyond the year 2000. *Infectious Disease Clinics of North America* 5(2):417–428.

Vujicic M, Zurn P, Diallo K, Dal Poz M. 2004. The role of wages in slowing the migration of health care professionals from developing countries. *Human Resources for Health* 2:3.

WHO (World Health Organization). 2004. *eHealth Report by the Secretariat.* Geneva, Switzerland: WHO. [Online]. Available: http://www.who.int/gb/ebwha/pdf_files/EB115/B115_39-en.pdf [accessed March 4, 2005].

Yudkin JS, Bayley O, Elnour S, Willott C, Miranda JJ. 2003. Introducing medical students to global health issues: A Bachelor of Science degree in international health. *Lancet* 362(9386):822–824.

Appendix A

Information Gathering Workshop Agendas

COMMITTEE ON THE OPTIONS FOR OVERSEAS PLACEMENT OF
U.S. HEALTH PROFESSIONALS

December 1, 2004
Lecture Room
National Academy of Sciences
2101 Constitution Avenue, NW
Washington, DC 20418

Introductions

1:00   Committee Chairman's Introduction
        Fitzhugh Mullan, Chair

1:10   Introductory Remarks
        *Mark Dybul, Assistant U.S. Global AIDS Coordinator and
        Chief Medical Officer,
        Office of the U.S. Global AIDS Coordinator*

Overview of Human Resource Health Care Needs, Challenges, and Solutions

1:30   Human Resource Needs for Scaling Up HIV Treatment and Prevention
        Barbara Stilwell, Department of Human Resources for Health, Cluster on Evidence and Information for Policy, WHO

1:50   HRH Challenges and Solutions in Low Resource HIV Areas
        Ummuro Adano, Management Sciences for Health

2:10   Quality of Care and Human Resources in HIV Health Care Programs
        James Heiby, Country Coordinator, USAID Bureau of Global Health

2:30   Panel Discussion
        Moderator: Fitzhugh Mullan

2:50   Break

Health Care Needs of Representative PEPFAR Countries

3:00   Zambia
        Gilbert Kombe, Abt Associates

3:15   Haiti
        Antoine Augustin, President and CEO MARCH Foundation

3:30   Vietnam
        Eric Krakauer, Director of the Vietnam–CDC–Harvard Medical School AIDS Partnership

3:45   Panel Discussion
        Moderator: Ronaldo Lima

4:05   Break

Lessons Learned from Large-Scale Training Efforts

4:15   Model of Training for Grass Roots Work in HIV
        King Holmes, University of Washington

4:35   How the U.S. Military Trains Medics
            Col. Maureen Coleman, (RTD) Commander of the 32nd
            Medical Brigade of the AMEDDC&S

4:55   International Medical Cooperation: Lessons from the Cuban
            Experience
            Gail A. Reed, International Director, Medical Education
            Cooperation with Cuba (MEDICC)

5:15   Panel Discussion
            Moderator: Jane Carter

5:35   Adjourn

                          December 2, 2004

            Nongovernmental Organization Models of Intervention:
            Lessons Learned from the Mobilization of Volunteers

8:30   Global Ministries
            Paul Dirdak, Deputy General Secretary, GBGM and UMCOR

8:50   International Medical Corps
            Ky Luu, Vice President, IMC

9:10   Potential Future Volunteers: Issues and Obstacles to Service
            Brian Palmer, AMSA

9:30   Mission Doctors Association
            Elise Frederick, Executive Director, MDA

9:50   Models of Care for Orphans and Vulnerable Children
            Karen Hein, past President of The William T. Grant
            Foundation

10:10   Panel Discussion
            Moderator: Gary Gunderson

10:30   Break

Governmental and Nongovernmental Models: Lessons Learned from the Deployment and Assignment of Volunteers and Paid Professionals

10:45   Peace Corps
            *Ronald Campbell, Country Director at Large, Office of the
            Director, Peace Corps*

11:00   USPHS-CDC
            *Mike St. Louis, Office of the Director,
            Global AIDS Program, CDC*

11:15   Twinning Centers and the HRSA Initiatives to Move the
            Domestic HIV Experience Internationally
            *Thurma McCann Goldman, HIV/AIDS Bureau Global
            Program, HRSA*

11:30   National Health Service Corps
            Don Weaver, Assistant Surgeon General, Director, NHSC

11:45   Volunteers for Prosperity, Freedom Corps
            Jack Hawkins, Director of Volunteers for Prosperity

12:00   Health Volunteers Overseas
            Nancy Kelly, Executive Director HVO

12:15   Panel Discussion
            Moderator: Michele Barry

12:35   Lunch

Building a Sustainable Health Care Workforce Through Training

1:35   HRH/HIV Opportunities: Equity and Sustainability
            *Holly Burkhalter, U.S. Policy Director, Physicians for Human
            Rights
            Eric Friedman, Health Action AIDS Policy Associate, PHR*

1:55   Training Kenyan Health Care Workers: An Academic
            Perspective
            *Fred Valentine, Director, Center for AIDS Research,
            NYU School of Medicine*

2:15   Partnering: University to University Training
          Robert Einterz, Assistant Dean and Director, IU-Moi Program

2:35   Panel Discussion
          Moderator: André-Jacques Neusy

2:55   Break

3:10   Academic Alliance for AIDS Care and Prevention in Africa
          Michael Scheld, UVA, Academic Alliance Foundation,
          co-director of the training programs

3:30   Ethical Issues in Foreign Health Workforce Assistance
          Programs
          Daniel Wikler, at Harvard School of Public Health

3:50   Educational Challenges in Building the Health Infrastructure
          to Combat HIV
          Barry Kistnasamy, Dean, Nelson Mandela School of Medicine

4:10   Panel Discussion
          Moderator: Fitzhugh Mullan

          **Summary of Presentations and Open Discussion with
          Guests, Speakers, and Committee**

4:30   Summary Comments: Main Speaker
          Harrison Spencer

4:45   Exchange of Ideas: Building an Overseas Health Care
          Workforce Model for HIV
          Fitzhugh Mullan

5:15   Adjourn

February 14, 2005
Room 101
Keck Building
500 Fifth Street, NW
Washington, DC 20001

9:30   Inventory of Sending Organizations and Lessons Learned
           John Shippee, Independent Consultant

10:00   Human Capacity Development in the 15 PEPFAR Countries
           Xingzhu Liu, PHRplus, Abt Associates Inc.

10:30   Telemedicine and Telehealth
           Holly Ladd, Satellife

11:00   The Charge to the Committee
           Joe O'Neill, Office of the U.S. Global AIDS Coordinator

11:30   Work within the PEPFAR Context
           Jim Smith, AIHA

12:00   Lunch

Appendix B

Ethical Issues in Foreign Health Workforce Assistance Programs

Presentation to the IOM Committee on December 2, 2004
Daniel Wikler, Ph.D.

Department of Population and International Health
Harvard School of Public Health

INTRODUCTION

Daniel Wikler is a professor of ethics in the Department of Population and International Health at Harvard School of Public Health. His presentation was designed to articulate ideas that were put forth during the course of the two-day meeting of the *Committee on the Options for Overseas Placement of U.S. Health Professionals*. He spoke about moral and logistical issues involved with sending U.S. health professionals overseas. These issues involved more questions than answers mainly because the ethical rules, guidelines, criteria, and evaluation would all depend on how the program is structured. Dr. Wikler began his presentation by describing two categories of ethical questions.

TESTIMONY

What I am doing here is more articulating ideas that have been in the air for a couple of days, rather than laying down any startling new ideas. First of all, wouldn't it be nice if we could say that the idea of a volunteer corps going all the way to Africa or to another very poor, struggling country to help with PEPFAR, help with relief of AIDS, doesn't need an ethical justification, doesn't need an ethics talk? If ever there was something that was obviously, self-evidently justified, this is it. It would be nice, but it is not true. So here are two categories of ethical questions. There are many more, but time doesn't allow.

The first has to do with questions that face this committee. They are questions in the design of the program. I don't think you can talk about ethical criteria unless you have some idea of what the program is. I have to confess, after two days, I really don't know what the program is meant to be. I have a feeling that I know where the committee is going. I have a feeling that [the funding organizations] had something else in mind. So what results, we will see.

I was thinking, what are the models? One model is the groups that do the emergency humanitarian intervention. There is an earthquake, and 75 aid groups all show up. They start pointing fingers at each other saying "We're the only sincere people here. You don't know what you are doing. You are just trying to increase your donations." They start fighting over who gets credit for what. Nothing is coordinated. There are major lapses. No one is keeping score. There is no one in charge, so there is no overall plan to make sure that all the bases are covered.

So what have you got? You have some really wonderful agencies that do wonderful work and try to keep tabs on each other as best they can. Their work is complicated by all kinds of other players who run around doing their own thing, sometimes tripping up the activities of the best agencies.

So that is not so great. It is not the model for this, obviously, partly because it is a very flawed model, and the better agencies all know it and they are trying to do something about it. But also these are very short-term interventions. As soon as you get things fixed up and stabilized, you are off to the next emergency. They happen because, usually, there has been a total breakdown.

The model for PEPFAR, of course, is totally different. You are basically thinking about stable regimes, with tragically stable or long-term patterns of suffering, and, presumably, one is there for the long haul. So that is not the right model.

What is the better model? Number two is what is already happening. We have heard for two days that there are a lot of people over there, a lot of Americans over there, working for different agencies, doing good work—God's work, as one might say. And bless them.

But this is sort of a bouquet of individual initiatives. Again, there is no one keeping score. There is no one in charge, no one who is trying to say, "Yes, we have covered all the main bases here," or, "I know you came over and you want to do this, but the real need is over here. Would you please do that?" There is nobody to report to and nobody to check off the needs and so on. So that is what is there.

Now, it is possible that what the [funders of PEPFAR] have in mind is that they would be something like that. Actually, what I heard was something less than that. They just want to encourage lots more of the shoots to come up.

The third one, which would be just great, would be to say, no, what we are really talking about here is how to prevent the complete breakdown of health systems, focusing on HIV/AIDS, but obviously with ramifications for other serious diseases. We are looking at the medium to long term. We want to make sure that the PEPFAR intervention is actually one that would enhance the other work, so we want to integrate PEPFAR with the other stuff that is happening. Either PEPFAR would be the integrator or ask WHO to play that role, or some other agency. The emphasis, being on the long term, would be on training. Moreover, there might be other aspects to intervention, beyond the focus on AIDS that this would also dovetail with.

That would just be wonderful. But I don't know what you are planning. The ethical rules, the ethical guidelines, the criteria, evaluation, and so on would all depend on which one of these you had in mind.

Let's look at some big-scale issues having to do with equity. These are not questions that face the individual volunteer. They face the people who are planning the system. We have this odd situation in which the United States is now talking about sending over planeloads of volunteers, and they will wave in the window to all those physicians coming from those very countries on their way to better jobs in the United States. What do you call this? You have volunteers, and you have brain drain. What happens when these are happening simultaneously?

I have just listed two views here. I am not going to endorse one of them. One would say that this is a sign of a serious inequity. It basically says that the fact that Africa is emptying out its health systems, both nurses and doctors, and they are coming to places like the United States is in part the fault of the rich countries. Why is that? Because we have jobs, in the state mental hospitals and less desirable jobs in general, that these people are filling—not always, but often. Why are they going empty? Why is it that people have to recruit abroad? Because those jobs aren't adequately recruited for or funded or whatever. We are producing lots of doctors, but our doctors have almost total discretion over where they practice, and we are not making those jobs attractive enough to lure them there.

So we sort of create a magnet, and sure enough, it draws people toward it. They are coming from these places where what we are offering is much better than what they would otherwise face. To that extent, the brain drain is partly our fault. So it is an inequity.

What it amounts to is a huge subsidy by the very poorest countries of the very richest. The NHS saves a caboodle by hiring the graduates of the Aga Khan medical school's nursing academy. The way it was described to me was that on graduation day, the nurses file out with their diplomas and there are tables set up with the Germans and the British and so on. They can take their pick. We don't recruit. We are not that gross. But there is complicity, too.

The other point of view, obviously, is that we didn't bring these people here. The way the world system works is, individuals get to go where they want. They choose to come here, which is not irrational. Since we don't recruit these doctors, we don't owe anybody any compensation. It is not a wrong that is done to them.

What hangs on this? If you have done a wrong to another country, you owe them something, basically. One question I would put to the committee is, Do you want to take a position on this? Do you want to address the fact that you are contemplating a volunteer corps at the same time that the very places that the volunteers would go to are sending their experts here and to England and so on?

If you don't address this, it seems to me that there is a blind spot in the report. It is a little bit other-worldly. That is the context in which this is being contemplated. At least to address it would show that you thought about it. I would think that would be a good idea. Then not only to address it, but to say what you actually think about it, which means debating it, would be even better.

So what should one say? Here are, again, three views, without any endorsement. The first one would say, keep your volunteers until we solve the brain-drain problem. Maybe we won't need volunteers if we could just keep the people we have. Help us with that. Help us raise the salaries so that people can earn a decent living, while providing medical care under unpleasant circumstances. Also don't make it so easy for them to come, and also fund your own system better so that you don't create these openings.

That one says, think twice before you engage in this volunteer effort.

The second view says, no, no, no, these are happening simultaneously, but they are otherwise unrelated. As a matter of fact, you could use the volunteers to help stem the brain drain, for example, by establishing long-term collegial relationships through twinning and so on. That might actually make it a more viable career to stay in some of these countries.

Also we could say that by providing the volunteers, we are partly compensating the countries for the subsidy that they are giving us by sending us their medical graduates.

The third one, which is sort of allied to the third view about what this program is about, is to say, yes, there are equity issues here, and there is a solution to the equity issues, which is that the United States will help go to the root causes of the brain drain and the critical lack of qualified personnel by shoring up the health systems. This PEPFAR effort is a step in that direction. But that means, of course, it has to be coordinated with and supplemented by other steps.

This is pretty obvious. One kind of ethical consideration is, is there anything that you might do in setting up a volunteer corps that would actually make things worse? Of course there is. There is a question about displacing the trade of existing practitioners. We know that food aid sometimes, even in humanitarian emergencies, has the net effect of increasing starvation, because when you give away food to people even in emergencies, neighboring farmers can't sell their produce. So, after a while, they will stop growing it, and the amount of food available may be actually less.

So with emergency food supplies, there is this kind of effect. Do we know whether this will occur with the use of volunteers?

Some emergency intervention agencies now insist that you never give away food. You charge for it, even if some people have to starve because they can't afford it, because it is too dangerous to do the opposite. What about this?

Is it possible that coming in with a vertical program, an AIDS-oriented program, would have the effect, since it is going to be well-funded, even though these may be volunteers, of drawing people away from primary care and from other kinds of treatment, which, in fact, may be more cost effective? After all, you don't really cure any AIDS patients. It is very expensive, year after year, and very labor intensive. Presumably, the people who are going to be drawn into this were not just idling. They were very busy before they would be drawn into it. What were they doing? Is what they are doing dispensable? Is it less cost effective than what they would be doing with the AIDS program, or are they just coming over because it is better-funded and offers all kinds of other opportunities? So that is a problem.

Finally, there is the question about abandonment. If PEPFAR comes in and people get antiretrovirals for a few years, and then the party is over and all the Americans go home—they have had a great experience, and they will never forget it. So good for them, but how about the people who were left behind? You could say, look, they would have died earlier if Americans hadn't come. But is that really the goal? Is that the only possibility? If there are other possibilities, then how does one exercise a responsible choice?

Let me switch over now, briefly, to some ethical issues facing volunteers. I don't think any of these will come as a surprise to you. First of all, having to do with selection of beneficiaries, setting priorities—there is an old distinction in moral philosophy between perfect and imperfect obligations. Perfect obligations are ones that you incur to specific individuals. I borrow your book; I owe you the book. If I give your book to somebody else who needs it or wants it, that doesn't fulfill my obligation. But there are imperfect obligations, like charity. I have an obligation to be charitable, but no one has a specific claim on my charity. I can more or less pick my beneficiary.

Which is it? What is PEPFAR? Is it the exercise of a perfect or an imperfect obligation? One of the differences might be that if it is imperfect, then any amount of good you do is fine; it is great. Right now, for example, we heard from all these programs that are selecting sites, that are going over; they are all doing good. Could you go to them and say, "I don't think you are a very upstanding outfit, because there is another place where you could have done even more good, and you didn't go there." You wouldn't think of saying that. It is amazing that they did as much as they did, and bravo for them.

PEPFAR, though, is a different order of magnitude here. I assume that we are talking about a larger and certainly more official governmental organization. So does it have an obligation, then, to select according to equity criteria as opposed to just treating whoever they want to treat, for whatever reasons? If they want to be equitable, they have to decide what would be equitable.

In situations like this—I think this is a criticism that has been made in regard to the WHO three-by-five program—this unremitting emphasis on the number of people treated basically blots out all equity considerations. If your only goal is to treat as many people as you can, then you will treat the people who are easiest to treat, easiest to get to. It means that you want your dollars, which will always be scarce, to go as far as they can.

That means if somebody can pay for themselves, you treat them for sure, because then you can use that money to treat somebody else. If somebody is out in the sticks and you have to bring some of these city doctors out there, then they go without treatment. If males are free to come into the clinic, but the females are basically locked up in the house, and it would be a big to-do if you wanted to go out there and combat this, so what if you have 70 percent males in your patient list?

So that is a question: To what extent should the volunteers go over there with a set of scruples, equity considerations, and an insistence that these are the rules that they have to play by? There are rules, or at least we hope there are. There are aspirations anyway. Should that be brought over to that environment?

You may find that there are some people there who share the same view about what equity is, and there are some who don't. In some countries, for example, small children just are not seen as important, whereas here sometimes they are seen as more important, and certainly with men and women. The fact that there is such stigma attached to AIDS means that this very disease marks somebody as less than worthy, as long as it is openly admitted that they have it.

These are the questions about expertise. Obviously, we are setting up a situation in which the American may go over with many more years of training, better training, than the host physician has. Then what do you do?

One hears often a plea for deference, for not trying to lord it over the host, and so on. There is a lot to be said for that. But on the next slide, what I have is basically an extended argument made to me by an African colleague, whom I respect very, very much. What he is trying to say, if you can read through this, is: Be nice. Don't make them feel bad. But don't, don't cede your ground. You are there to raise the standards. Never lose sight of that. Do everything you can to dance around the fact that you know and they don't know, but don't give up. If it doesn't work the first time, try it again. He had various strategies for doing it. What the volunteers go there for and what PEPFAR is [there] for may be somewhat different. As we heard before, there are all kinds of motives for people to go over. If they have different motives, we don't know what they will do when they get there.

Should there be limits on what they do? Should we say that we don't really care what else they do, as long as they do their treating, and if they are there to do something else, go for it? Or should you say, look, we are there for AIDS; the rest of the stuff you can do on some other trip to Africa?

With public–private partnerships, you have the additional consideration that some of your private partners may have commercial motives. They may be pursuing those. They may be using your cover as a way of legitimizing them. So what do you do about that? It is a chronic problem, of course.

Finally, I was wondering whether it would be useful for the committee to say that there should be some ethical constraints, some ground rules that govern basically all aspects of the program. It is very hard to draw these things up without being vapid. The ideal is something that is general enough so that you don't come up with immediate counter-examples, but specific enough so that it has some actual force. A few times, somebody actually achieves these.

Just thinking this through with some colleagues, here are a few candidates. I am not necessarily endorsing any of these, and certainly not this set of six. But they are examples of what these rules could look like:

- Benefit to the host country is the fundamental criterion of adequacy.
- Capacity-building over the medium and long term is the primary goal.
- The work of a PEPFAR volunteer corps should be coordinated with other initiatives to allocate resources rationally.
- Needs are defined by host countries.
- Standard of care is defined by the needs of the host country.
- Volunteers should respect hosts values but must be governed by their own values, including equity in selection of patients.

I think when one comes up with the magic formula, something that has the right degree of bite and generality, it is very, very useful, because it gives you a benchmark against which later infractions or deviations can be held to account.

Appendix C

Assessing the Human Resource Need for Expanding HIV/AIDS Services in the 15 PEPFAR Focus Countries

Gilbert Kombe, Xingzhu Liu, Nancy Pielemeier,
Catherine Decker

Abt Associates

BACKGROUND

There is broad recognition that human capacity is a critical constraint in scaling up HIV/AIDS services in low-resource countries. Difficulties in producing and retaining a sufficient number of health workers is not a new problem, but the sheer magnitude of the HIV/AIDS epidemic and its impact on human resources (HR)[1] through an array of supply and demand-side factors has made the problem worse (Smith, 2004). For example, in sub-Saharan Africa, both budgetary stringency and fiscal economic crises have reduced the governments' ability to attract and train health workers, as well as to retain them and maintain their morale. Studies indicate that the numbers of trained health workers in many low resource areas remain insufficient and currently many such settings are experiencing serious scarcities of almost all cadres due to economic and fiscal difficulties (USAID, 2003). According to the World Health Organization (WHO), about 100,000 health workers globally need to be trained in order to reach the target to deliver antiretroviral therapy (ART) to 3 million people. These health workers include those involved in managing and delivering antiretroviral treatment services, those working on testing and counseling, and community treatment supporters assisting people living with HIV/AIDS who are receiving medication (WHO, 2003).

---

[1]The term "human resource" is interchangeably used with "health care workers," "health workers," and "providers."

There are many reasons why the United States Government (USG) should invest in understanding the magnitude and complexity of HR issues in the 15 focus countries. First, these countries account for more than 50 percent of all global infections and nearly 75 percent of all HIV infections in Sub-Saharan Africa. It is estimated that without a significantly expanded response to the epidemic, more people will become infected in the next few years. Second, there is compelling evidence from published and unpublished reports that the 15 countries studied have a critical shortage of human resource stock. The current ratio of key health workers to population in each country is not encouraging. According to the latest available information, 7 of the 15 countries have a ratio less than one doctor to 5,000 and 6 of them have a ratio below one nurse to 2,000 inhabitants as shown in Table C-1. These ratios are well below the WHO recommended minimum standard of one doctor per 5,000 inhabitants and one nurse per 500 population. Third, understanding the number of available health care workers, their skill mix, training needs, and the distribution of such personnel is essential in planning a USG response to fill in HR gaps through allocation of appropriate resources. This information can also be of critical value to countries themselves in developing appropriate strategies to address the HR problems to improve their overall health systems. As the President Emergency Plan for AIDS Relief (PEPFAR) countries begin to scale up HIV/AIDS activities, increased attention should focus on identifying and addressing these HR constraints.

The objective of this paper is to provide broad estimates on the quantity and mix of human resources needed to deliver full HIV/AIDS services in PEPFAR countries. The paper is organized in the following manner. First, the paper presents the methodological approach used in the analysis. Second, it presents specific findings on the current and projected future HR stocks, projects the HR needs to provide full HIV/AIDS services[2] under PEPFAR targets, and identifies the gaps. Finally, it recommends strategies to fill these HR gaps, discusses policy implications and the way forward.

METHODOLOGICAL APPROACH

A comprehensive desktop review of published and unpublished documents was conducted to obtain information on human resources in the 15

---

[2]The term "full HIV/AIDS services" used here refers to antiretroviral therapy (ART), voluntary counseling and testing (VCT), prevention of mother-to-child transmission (PMTCT) and treatment of opportunistic infections (OIs). It excludes activities such as care of orphans and vulnerable children, information education and communication, condom distribution, management information systems, etc.

TABLE C-1 Basic HIV/AIDS Indices and Human Resource Status in the 15 PEPFAR Focus Countries

Country	Population (year)		Population with HIV (15–49)[b]	HIV Prevalence (15–49) %[b]
Botswana	1,646,640	(1999)[a]	270,000	37.3
Cote d'Ivoire	14,685,000	(1996)[d]	530,000	7.0
Ethiopia	68,613,470	(2003)[a]	1,400,000	4.4
Kenya	27,390,000	(1995)[d]	1,100,000	6.7
Mozambique	17,691,000	(2000)[a]	1,200,000	12.2
Namibia	1,750,000	(1997)[d]	200,000	21.3
Nigeria	126,910,000	(2000)[a]	3,300,000	5.4
Rwanda	8,163,000	(2002)[a]	230,000	5.1
South Africa	44,812,420	(2001)[a]	5,100,000	21.5
Tanzania	35,181,300	(2002)[a]	1,500,000	8.8
Uganda	24,600,000	(2002)[a]	450,000	4.1
Zambia	10,402,960	(2003)[a]	830,000	24.6
Haiti	7,797,000	(1998)[d]	260,000	5.6
Guyana	759,000	(2000)[a]	11,000	2.5
Vietnam	79,492,930	(2001)[a]	200,000	0.4

[a]World Development Indicators Database, World Bank (http://devdata.worldbank.org/dataquery/).
[b]2004 Report on the Global AIDS Epidemic, UNAIDS.

PEPFAR focus countries. The latest available data were collected from various databases and documents from sources such as UNAIDS, WHO, World Bank, etc. Information was also supplemented by country assessments conducted by the Partners for Health Reform*plus* Project and other collaborating agencies. The WHO online Global Atlas of the Health Workforce was the primary source of data on the current HR stock for each country by year and by profession.[3]

In making HR projections, a number of key assumptions were applied. We discuss five assumptions that have the most impact on human resource

---

[3]This database has the latest available data on health personnel including doctors and nurses for all PEPFAR countries. Some statistics were found on pharmacists and midwives but not for all 15 countries. Personnel such as lab technicians and counselors were not included. Based on a previous conversation with the database manager, for some countries, both public and private sector data are included, although it is unclear how consistently private sector HR data are included across countries.

Total Number of Doctors (year)[c]	Doctor per Population Ratio	Total Number of Nurses (year)[c]	Nurse per Population Ratio
488 (1999)	3,374	4090 (1999)	403
1,322 (1996)	11,108	6,785 (1996)	2,164
1,162 (2003)	59,048	14,123 (2003)	4,858
3,616 (1995)	7,575	24,679 (1995)	1,110
435 (2000)	40,669	5,078 (2000)	3,484
516 (1997)	3,392	4,978 (1997)	352
30,885 (2000)	4,109	154,000 (2003)	824
155 (2002)	52,665	1,745 (2002)	4,678
30,740 (2001)	1,458	172,338 (2001)	260
822 (2002)	42,800	13,292 (2002)	2,647
1,175 (2002)	20,936	2,200 (2002)	11,182
756 (2003)	13,761	10,558 (2003)	985
1,949 (1998)	4,001	834 (1998)	9,349
366 (2000)	2,074	1,738 (2000)	437
42,327 (2001)	1,878	59,201 (2001)	1,343

[c]All statistics come from WHO online Global Atlas of the Health Workforce (www.who.int/ GlobalAtlas/home.asp) except data on Ethiopia ("The Human and Financial Resource Requirements for Scaling Up HIV/AIDS Services in Ethiopia." Kombe et al. February 2005. PHRplus), ("Health Manpower Situation in Nigeria: Nigeria, 1995-2000." Health Manpower Registration Councils/Boards) and Zambia.

[d]"Human Resources for Health: Overcoming the Crisis." Joint Learning Initiative, 2004.

needs for providing full HIV/AIDS services. First, with regard to ART, individual country targets for ART were estimated by determining country weights based on the number of infected adults in the individual country divided by the total number of infected adults in all 15 countries. This number was then multiplied by 2 million to obtain the individual country target for ART. Second, we assumed that all patients not receiving ART would need OI care. Therefore, OI targets were estimated by subtracting the ART target from the estimated number of patients eligible for ART.

Third, it is assumed that VCT and PMTCT will be gateways to HAART in a manner characterized by certain key ratios. It is assumed here that the diagnosis rate of HIV-positive individuals is twice the country-specific prevalence rate (to account for self-selection). Also, it is assumed that 20 percent of those identified as HIV positive individuals will be clinically eligible as suggested under the PEPFAR Initiative. Fourth, we estimated the HR need by multiplying the number of encounters per patient by the time needed per encounter by the size of target population. The total time is then converted into person-year by considering the number of working days per year (180), and the number of effective working hours (6),[4] and the average share of provider's time used for HIV services (50 percent).[5] We then multiply the number of person-years by (a) the number of people in need of HIV/AIDS services and (b) the PEPFAR target population.

The fifth assumption deals with estimating projected HR growth over the next 5 years. The annual growth rate of the HR stock of each country over the next 5 years is assumed to be equivalent to the annual growth rate of the past 5 years. The aggregate growth rate is the weighted average of the growth rates of individual countries—estimated at 4.5 percent.

MAIN FINDINGS

Five main findings can be drawn from this paper. First, as shown in Table C-2, the total human resource stock available in 2004 is estimated at 566,580. This number does not include community health workers, counselors, and social workers due to lack of data. Nurses and midwives[6] make up the majority (74 percent) followed by doctors (21 percent), and pharmacists (5 percent). Applying the 2004 baseline data and assuming that existing conditions are not going to change, the projected growth in the total number of health workers will increase from 566,580 in 2004 to 592,076 in 2008 at an annual rate of approximately 4.5 percent. This increase is primarily driven by Nigeria, South Africa, and Vietnam, all countries with large populations and high personnel totals. Meanwhile, countries like Tanzania and Uganda will see a decrease in the total HR stock. The remaining 10 PEPFAR countries will have a minimal growth in the next 4 years.

Second, to provide full HIV/AIDS services to all eligible patients, the total human resource need is about 78,360 in 2004, rising to 95,246 in 2008. To reach PEPFAR targets, the total human resource need is about 11,232 in 2004, but by 2008, this figure will increase to 56,146 due to the planned scale-up of PEPFAR funded programs (see Table C-3 for country specific data). It must be noted that PEPFAR needs are a subset of the total number of health workers to provide full HIV/AID services.

Third, the question of how many health workers have been trained in the 15 PEPFAR countries has been a subject of debate by many health planners. It is estimated that on average 10 percent of the health workers

---

[4]Based on workforce study in Zambia, on average a doctor spends approximately 18.5 minutes per visit (average of 22 minutes for the initial visit and 15 minutes for follow-up visits) with a patient on ART (Huddart et al. 2004).

[5]Therefore, full time equivalent (FTE) requirements are half those presented below.

[6]Nurses and midwives are categorized together in this study.

TABLE C-2 Current and Projected Human Resource Stock in the 15 PEPFAR Focus Countries

Gross Human Resource Stock by Type	Available in: 2004	2005	2006	2007	2008
Doctors	117,523	123,230	129,265	135,649	142,403
Nurses	419,906	424,247	429,246	434,864	441,071
Pharmacists	29,151	29,930	30,755	31,604	32,484
Total	566,580	577,407	589,266	602,117	615,958
Estimated number of health workers trained in HIV care	56, 658	57,245	57,865	58,518	59,208

including doctors, nurses and pharmacists have already been trained in full HIV/AIDS service provision in each of the countries. Based on this assumption, the number of available staff trained to provide HIV/AIDS services is 10 percent of the figures shown in Table C-2, increasing from 56,658 to 59,208 between 2004 and 2008 respectively. There has also been a lot of debate on how many health workers are needed to reach the PEPFAR goals of 2 million people on ART, preventing 7 million infections, and providing care to 10 million orphans and vulnerable children. Under the PEPFAR initiative, in 2005, the total number of trained health workers needed to reach PEPFAR targets is approximately 4,431.[7] This number will almost double in 2006 to roughly 8,676.

Fourth, we explore the issue of "human resource gap" by comparing the trained health workers with estimated HR needs over the next 4 years. The HR gap is an indication of the severity of human resources shortages. To put this into context, the magnitude of HR Gap is illustrated for doctors, nurses and pharmacists. As shown in Figure C-1, in 2004 the number of trained doctors falls well short of those needed to treat all patients eligible for HIV services.

The gap is widest for pharmacists, followed by doctors, with nurses showing a gap of only 10 percent (having 41,991 trained out of 46,635 needed). In all three cases the gap widens as time goes by, resulting in insufficient numbers of trained doctors and pharmacists for the provision of PEPFAR services in 2008. This human resource gap exists for both

---

[7]Note that the HR gap to reach the PEPFAR targets is a subset of the gap to reach all of those in need.

TABLE C-3 Estimated Total of Key Health Workers Needed to Deliver
Health Services in the 15 PEPFAR Focus Countries

Country	Staff Type	2004 Available	PEPFAR Needed
Botswana	Doctors	488	66
	Nurses	4,090	66
	Pharmacists	160	35
Cote d'Ivoire	Doctors	1,322	89
	Nurses	6,785	200
	Pharmacists	378	46
Ethiopia	Doctors	1,971	232
	Nurses	4,160	703
	Pharmacists	95	118
Kenya	Doctors	3,616	215
	Nurses	24,679	419
	Pharmacists	1,370	112
Mozambique	Doctors	435	210
	Nurses	5,078	433
	Pharmacists	419	108
Namibia	Doctors	516	34
	Nurses	4,978	44
	Pharmacists	149	17
Nigeria	Doctors	30,885	580
	Nurses	108,230	1,537
	Pharmacists	8,642	300
Rwanda	Doctors	155	41
	Nurses	1,745	91
	Pharmacists	11	21
South Africa	Doctors	30,740	872
	Nurses	172,338	1,371
	Pharmacists	10,742	453
Tanzania	Doctors	822	269
	Nurses	13,292	540
	Pharmacists	365	140
Uganda	Doctors	1,175	103
	Nurses	2,200	154
	Pharmacists	125	55

2006		2008	
Available	PEPFAR Needed	Available	PEPFAR Needed
551	197	622	329
4,451	197	4,844	329
173	106	188	177
1,444	268	1,577	447
7,409	601	8,091	1,002
413	138	451	230
2,167	695	2,383	1,159
4,176	2,109	4,192	3,516
106	354	119	589
3,949	646	4,312	1,076
26,950	1,256	29,430	2,094
1,496	337	1,634	562
529	629	643	1,048
5,162	1,298	5,247	2,163
434	323	449	538
563	102	615	169
5,436	132	5,936	219
163	52	178	87
35,911	1,739	41,755	2,898
108,230	4,610	108,230	7,684
8,642	599	8,642	1,498
169	123	185	204
1,906	274	2,081	457
12	63	13	105
33,556	2,616	36,630	4,361
172,338	4,112	172,338	6,853
11,189	1,358	11,655	2,264
727	808	643	1,347
9,696	1,619	7,073	2,698
323	419	285	698
1,283	310	1,401	517
1,514	461	1,043	768
131	165	143	275

continued

TABLE C-3 Continued

Country	Staff Type	2004 Available	PEPFAR Needed
Zambia	Doctors	756	152
	Nurses	10,558	242
	Pharmacists	75	79
Haiti	Doctors	1,949	44
	Nurses	834	109
	Pharmacists	557	23
Guyana	Doctors	366	2
	Nurses	1,738	6
	Pharmacists	86	1
Vietnam	Doctors	42,327	31
	Nurses	59,201	853
	Pharmacists	5,977	16

reaching all those in need and reaching the PEPFAR targets. The current trained HR stock is not enough to provide full HIV/AIDS services to all those in need.

To further illustrate this HR gap, we analyzed the gap for doctors across the 15 countries. As shown in Box C-1, the 15 countries were divided into six categories according to the adult HIV prevalence rate (for those aged 15–49) and doctor gap (total need for doctors *divided by* total stock of doctors) *multiplied by* 100 to give percentage). The HR gap was divided into three groups: severe, moderate and low. Prevalence was divided into high (greater than 6 percent) and low (less than 6 percent).

An initial review of the HR gap for doctors points towards an association between the gap of a country and its HIV prevalence rate. First, none of the countries with high HR gaps have low HIV prevalence rates. Second, all of the low prevalence countries are either low or medium HR gap countries.

In general, the estimated HR gap in many countries will increase along with the scaling-up of PEPFAR programs year by year. Countries such as Cote D'Ivoire, Vietnam, and Guyana have only a modest doctor gap, while Tanzania, Mozambique, Botswana, and Zambia have large gaps. It is vital to point out that in the latter countries, the provision of HIV/AIDS services will absorb more than 100 percent of the available stock because the total doctor need is larger than the available stock. Namibia, Ethiopia, Rwanda, Uganda and Kenya have medium gaps and are expected to absorb over 50

2006		2008	
Available	PEPFAR Needed	Available	PEPFAR Needed
783	455	810	758
10,558	726	10,558	1,210
75	236	75	393
2,128	133	2,224	222
911	327	952	545
608	69	636	115
400	6	436	10
1,898	17	2,073	29
94	3	103	5
45,105	92	48,066	153
59,201	2,560	59,201	4,266
6,096	47	6,217	79

percent of the doctor stock for the provision of HIV/AIDS services. In Cote d'Ivoire and South Africa where the gap is low and the prevalence rate is high the provision of HIV/AIDS services will utilize less than 50 percent of the HR stock because they have a large HR stock. Finally, countries with a low HR gap and a low prevalence rate, such as Guyana, Haiti, Nigeria, and Vietnam will also absorb less than 50 percent of HR stock for the provision of HIV/AIDS services.

Finally, the projected gaps in trained HIV/AIDS personnel, in particular for doctors, lead to the fifth finding. Countries need to mobilize a large number of master trainers to train health workers on HIV/AIDS care. The need for master trainers is estimated in 2 parts. First, we consider the need to train enough trainees to provide full HIV/AIDS services to all eligible patients. In 2005, the 15 countries will need approximately 3,067 master trainers.[8] These trainers will include 1,141 doctors, 1,209 nurses, and 717 pharmacists, as shown in Table C-4. Second, we focus on the master trainers needed under the PEPFAR Initiative. Our analysis indicates that in 2005, the total need for master trainers for PEPFAR is 354,[9] which increases to 1629 (580 doctors, 631 nurses, and 418 pharmacists) by 2008.

---

[8]We assumed that 1 master trainer trains between 10–15 trainees, an average of 12.5. This assumption was made based on previous studies in Zambia, Nigeria, and Ethiopia (Kombe, 2003; 2004).

[9]Please note this is a subset of the need for master trainers to reach all those in need.

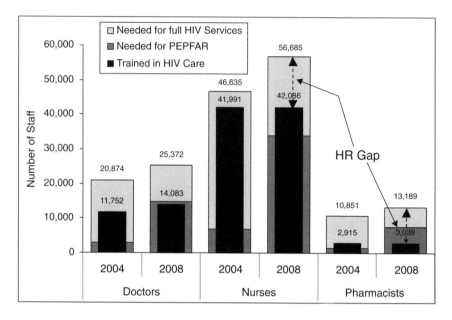

FIGURE C-1 Human resource gap for doctors, nurses (including midwives), and pharmacists.

SENSITIVITY ANALYSIS

A sensitivity analysis was performed to determine the extent to which the human resources vary along with the variation in the assumed percentage of health worker's time used for HIV/AIDS services. The analysis was performed by changing the percentage share between a minimum of 25 percent and a maximum of 75 percent, with 50 percent as the average.[10] For example, if the percentage share of providers' time used for HIV/AIDS services decreases from 50 percent to 25 percent, the estimated HR gap (PEPFAR HR need minus HIV/AIDS trained HR) increases from 20,361 to 63,725, more than triple as shown in Table C-5.

LIMITATIONS OF THE STUDY

This review and analysis has several limitations. First, the availability and reliability of the HR data was not consistent across the 15 PEPFAR

---

[10]Note that this does not change the FTE requirements, but rather the number of health workers who need to be trained.

BOX C-1
Categorization of Countries According to the Level of
Prevalence and Doctors' Gap[a]

	HIV Prevalence	
Doctor Gap (total need for doctors/total stock of doctors)[a] 100%	High Adult HIV/AIDS Prevalence (more than 6%)	Low Adult HIV/AIDS Prevalence (less than 6%)
Severe (>100%)	Tanzania Mozambique Botswana Zambia	
Moderate (50-100%)	Namibia Kenya	Ethiopia Rwanda Uganda
Low (<50%)	Cote d'Ivoire South Africa	Guyana Haiti Nigeria Vietnam

[a]Assumption that 50 percent of HR time is used for HIV/AIDS services

countries. It is not known whether all the data collected from the WHO online Global Atlas of the Health Workforce includes the private sector providers. Health personnel such as laboratory technicians and counselors are excluded from this analysis due to the lack of data.

Second, in some countries like Guyana and Rwanda, only 1 point of data was available, reducing the power of projection. Similarly, data on the numbers of deaths, retirements, emigrants, immigrants, staff turnovers, new graduates, etc. needed to estimate the decrease or increase of stock were not available, leading to the assumption that the change in the next 4 years will follow the pattern of the past 5 years (which may not be accurate).

Third, this lack of available data and time constraint restricted the opportunity for a detailed country level analysis. Therefore, it is extremely important to point out that all analyses are considered to be approximations and can only be used broadly for the development of an overall human resource capacity building strategy, rather than for country level planning. Fourth, key assumptions (e.g., time share between HIV/AIDS with non-HIV/AIDS services) have a significant impact on HR gap estimates. Finally, it must also be noted that the analysis is restricted to na-

TABLE C-4 Estimated Need for Master Trainers in the 15 PEPFAR Focus Countries

	2004	2005	2006	2007	2008
Need for Master Trainers to Provide full HIV/AIDS Services to all Eligible Patients					
Doctors	1,058	1,141	1,227	1,318	1,413
Nurses	1,082	1,209	1,342	1,482	1,631
Pharmacists	674	717	762	809	859
Total	2,814	3,067	3,331	3,609	3,903
Need for Master Trainers to Reach PEPFAR Targets					
Doctors	41	136	249	395	580
Nurses	25	126	269	441	631
Pharmacists	35	92	177	297	418
Total	101	354	695	1,133	1,629

TABLE C-5 Sensitivity Analysis of Human Resource Gap in the 15 PEPFAR Focus Countries in 2009

	25% of Health Worker's Time Used for HIV Services	50% of Health Worker's Time Used for HIV Services	75% of Health Worker's Time Used for HIV Services
Number of Trained Health Workers Needed to Provide PEPFAR Services			
Doctors	21,591	7,244	3,578
Nurses	29,376	7,893	4,033
Pharmacists	12,758	5,224	2,713
Total	63,725	20,361	10,324
Number of Trained Health Workers Needed to Provide Full HIV/AIDS Services to all in Need			
Doctors	42,726	17,662	9,325
Nurses	71,452	20,385	9,477
Pharmacists	23,798	10,740	6,400
Total	137,976	48,787	25,202

tional level because of data limitations on distribution of health workers between rural and urban settings.

DISCUSSION

Policy Implications of the Findings

Numerous studies have identified the major policy and program priorities needed to address the human resource gap in low resource countries, particularly those highly impacted by HIV/AIDS (JLI, 2004). The solutions focus on strategies to improve recruitment, retraining, retention and redeployment of health personnel. This analysis focuses primarily on the first 2 solutions: recruitment, or increasing the total stock of human resources, and retraining of existing personnel to deliver priority HIV/AIDS services. This is not meant to imply that retention and redeployment, or the re-engineering of tasks among various categories of health personnel, are not critical to address the AIDS epidemic, as well as to address the overall crisis in human resources for health (HRH). However, the scope of this study and the limitations of available data limit our ability to draw firm conclusions on these strategic options beyond endorsing others' calls to identify strategies to improve health worker salaries and incentives to increase retention, and to identify alternative personnel mixes to provide HIV/AIDS services.

The data limitations faced in this study do raise an issue of first order priority, noted also by similar studies (JLI, 2004; Martineau, 2004), that there is an urgent need for investment in databases and monitoring systems for human resources for health. The data available are insufficient, as illustrated by the lack of information on key categories of personnel, such as laboratory technicians and counselors, and therefore likely undercounting the total stock. It is highly likely that the countries that appear from this analysis to have the lowest human resource gap are precisely the countries that are losing the highest numbers of health personnel to international migration.

Notwithstanding the limitations of the data on which this analysis is based, there are a number of emerging implications for human resource policy development, which are likely to persist even when more precise human resource data become available. This analysis pinpoints the variation in the human resource gap across PEPFAR countries, based on HIV prevalence level, as well as on the relative scarcity of HRH. The program priorities vary slightly according to classification of countries within these dimensions; however, all PEPFAR countries need to focus on training of existing personnel, and most, if not all, PEPFAR countries need to focus on retaining and expanding the total HRH stock.

Conclusion

It is apparent that the HRH gap is a major constraint for both providing full coverage for HIV/AIDS services and reaching PEPFAR targets. The fact that many countries have a smaller stock of doctors and pharmacists than nurses calls for targeted strategies to address the shortage. Efforts should also be made to continue training large numbers of nurses and midwives to keep pace with migration and to fill the huge demand for nurses. If HRH capacity strategies are not implemented at the early stages of the PEPFAR program, the constraint will be more severe and plans to scale up will prove more difficult. Countries and development partners should define the role of donor assistance in training of trainers, and determine under what circumstances donors should be involved in direct training of staff and direct delivery of care in the short, medium, and long term, in order to meet both short-term PEPFAR goals, as well as longer term goals to provide sustained services to the affected population.

Second, each country should develop a national human resource for health plan. As recommended by the JLI, these plans should guide enhanced investments in human resources through appropriate education, deployment, and retention.

Third, development partners should work together under the guidance of the host government and within the country's national human resource plan to support both basic training of additional recruits, as well as in-service training of existing personnel, to meet the growing requirements for HRH for HIV/AIDS services.

The Way Forward

It is clear from the analysis that the way forward should focus on building innovative and sustainable strategies to address HRH in the 15 countries. Governments and donors should design and implement strategies for training the existing human resources for HIV/AIDS services. They should invest in conducting country specific HRH assessments and develop HRH plans according to specific country need. Furthermore, they should improve databases and monitoring systems for human resource for health.

REFERENCES

Health Manpower Registration Councils/Boards. 2001. *Health Manpower Situation in Nigeria: 1995–2000.*

Huddart J, Lyons JV, Furth R. 2004. *The Zambia HIV/AIDS Workforce Study: Preparing for Scale-Up.* [Online]. Available: http://www.qaproject.org/pubs/PDFs/ORMZambia Workforce1.pdf [accessed February 8, 2005].

JLI (Joint Learning Initiative). 2004. *Human Resources for Health: Overcoming the Crisis.* [Online]. http://www.globalhealthtrust.org/report/Human_Resources_for_Health.pdf [accessed February 9, 2005].

Kombe G, Smith O. 2003. *The Costs of Anti-Retroviral Treatment in Zambia.* [Online]. Available: http://www.phrplus.org/Pubs/Tech029_fin.pdf [accessed February 8, 2005].

Kombe G, Galaty D, Gadhia R, Decker C. 2005. *The Human and Financial Resource Requirements for Scaling Up HIV/AIDS Services in Ethiopia.* [Online]. Available: http://www.phrplus.org/Pubs/Tech059_fin.pdf [accessed February 18, 2005].

Kombe G, Galaty D, Nwagbara C. 2004. *Scaling Up Antiretroviral Treatment in the Public Sector in Nigeria: A Comprehensive Analysis of Resource Requirements.* [Online]. Available: http://www.phrplus.org/Pubs/Tech037_fin.pdf [accessed February 8, 2005].

Martineau T, 2004. *Staffing Options for Emergency HIV/AIDS programs.* Unpublished draft.

Smith O. 2004. Human resource requirements for scaling up antiretroviral therapy in low resource countries. In *Scaling Up Treatment in the Global AIDS Pandemic.* Washington, DC: The National Academies Press. Pp 292–308.

UNAIDS. 2004. *2004 Report on the Global AIDS Epidemic.* [Online]. Available: http://www.unaids.org/bangkok2004/report_pdf.html [accessed February 7, 2004].

USAID (U.S. Agency for International Development). 2003. *The Health Sector Human Resource Crisis in Africa: An Issues Paper.* [Online]. Available: http://www.aed.org/ToolsandPublications/upload/healthsector.pdf [accessed February 18, 2005].

WHO (World Health Organization). 2003. *Human Capacity-Building Plan for Scaling Up HIV/AIDS Treatment.* Geneva, Switzerland: World Health Organization.

WHO. 2004. *WHO Online Global Atlas for Health Workers* [Online]. Available: www.who.int/GlobalAtlas/home.asp [accessed February 7, 2005].

World Bank. 2004. *World Development Indicators Database.* [Online]. Available: http://www.worldbank.org/data/dataquery.html [accessed February 7, 2005].

Appendix D

U.S. Organizational Experience with Volunteer Health Programs

John Shippee

Shippee Consulting

INTRODUCTION

For the purpose of this paper, representatives from U.S. organizations who send volunteers to work overseas in health programs were surveyed. The survey was intended as a preliminary exploration of the experience of such organizations in sending volunteer health professionals to resource poor countries. Special attention was given to organizations deploying volunteers to work in HIV/AIDS. For several reasons, this effort must be considered a preliminary study that points (perhaps strongly) in certain directions, rather than an authoritative undertaking.

More than 80 organizations were considered for inclusion, and 66 were contacted primarily through e-mail. A survey and cover letter from the investigator and study director were emailed to each participant and followed up with a telephone call from the investigator. Most surveys were completed as telephone interviews. Of the 66 organizations contacted, 31 completed the full survey; and 30 of the 31 organizations completing the survey send volunteer medical professionals. Responses to the survey have been compiled for this report.

The organizations contacted and surveyed fell into the eight categories as outlined in Table D-1.

As measured by their overall annual budgets (gifts in kind excluded), the respondents ranged from small missionary organizations annually funded at less than $200,000 to large international organizations that have global budgets of roughly $1.5 billion. Many of these organizations have dedicated funding for the "battle against HIV/AIDS."

TABLE D-1 Organizations by Category

Organization Type	Number Contacted	Number Completing Surveys	Number Sending Medical Professionals
University Programs	11	9	9
General Development Organizations (Secular)	12	2	2
General Development Organizations (Faith-Based)	12	4	4
General Volunteer Organizations (Secular)	1	1	1
General Volunteer Organizations (Faith-Based)	9	5	5
Medical and Medical Volunteer Organizations (Secular)	7	6	6
Medical and Medical Volunteer Organizations (Faith-based)	10	2	2
HIV/AIDS Organizations	4	2	1
TOTAL	66	31	30

The lengths of service for volunteers in each organization varied from a few weeks to years. Renewable multiyear agreements with formalized contracts were available for some missionary organizations and university medical faculties. For the purpose of this study, organizations were divided into short (under 2 months), medium (2 to 6 months), and long-term volunteer (longer than 6 month) assignments.

Compensation by these organizations to medical professionals also varied. This study included but was not limited to organizations that offered no remuneration or subsistence level stipends.

PARTNERING CHALLENGES CITED BY RESPONDENTS

Organizational and Interorganizational Issues

Respondents identified a number of challenges to long-term partnering. This category includes obstacles to cooperation that can arise as a result of differences in organizational structure, expectations, and cultures between partnering organizations.

National and Local Obstacles

Cited challenges include overly onerous national and local governmental bureaucracy; difficulty obtaining in-country work permits; and trouble understanding complex local medical licensing regulations. Other reported barriers were the inability to cash traveler's checks and use credit cards.

International Obstacles

Less frequently, respondents reported difficulty in following the rules and procedures of their own and/or other international agencies and governments. These included such matters as difficulties in transferring funds to host and partner organizations; insistence on introducing antiretroviral therapy into treatment programs already using other regimens; and "overevaluation" that could mean having to carry out several different evaluations by related sponsoring agencies assessing essentially the same organizational procedures.

Communication Challenges

Communication obstacles in international partnership arrangements can take a variety of forms. Examples include lack of clarity regarding volunteer expectations (doctors expecting to focus on direct care being asked to administer programs); differences in the belief of how best to carry out certain administrative procedures; unmet expectations regarding volunteers' working or living conditions; and simple procedural misunderstandings between international partners.

Another communication obstacle—spoken or unspoken—can be the perceived or real arrogance or unwillingness to communicate on the part of very large organizations. One respondent cited this as an impediment and described their organization's efforts (not always fully successful) to overcome this communication obstacle with their often much smaller partners.

Lack of Mutual Clarity Regarding Project Goals and Expectations

Closely related to poor communication was the frequently cited challenge involving a lack of mutual clarity regarding goals and expectations. Each party in a partnership (including volunteers who are helping to implement it) needs to have a clear and explicit understanding of the extent and limitations of their mission, objectives, and responsibilities. Many problems can arise when this is not clearly stated at the beginning of a partnership and redefined as new situations arise. For example, considerable disruption can ensue if an international partner cannot provide promised funding in a timely manner or local partners have exaggerated expectations of the international partner's funding capabilities. Similarly, international volunteers (or employees) expecting to find Western medical supplies and efficient documentation systems in developing countries will likely find major frustrations with their host organization's working environment. This difficulty is compounded in partnering situations in which the international organization and local partners enter into agreements that do not take into account the very different "health worlds" or medical cultures from which each come.

Lack of Local Supervision of Volunteers

Volunteers and particularly those lacking relevant international experience, will require reliable local supervision, support, and orientation to situations and circumstances. Volunteers who do not have proper supervision may feel isolated, unable to use their skills, and frustrated in their work. Local partners, on the other hand, may simply not have the time (or in some cases, the skills) to provide a sufficient level of supervision and orientation needed for most international volunteers.

Local Partner Dependency

Partnerships are often constrained by funding. When the funding cycle ends, new sources are needed to sustain a long-term relationship. Creating false expectations that funding will continue without time limitations can leave a partner organization in a precarious situation, which is particularly dangerous in HIV/AIDS treatment partnerships. Once a support level for specific HIV/AIDS activities (i.e., ARV provision, prevention education, or orphan support) has been established, it must be maintained either nationally, internationally, or locally or else consequences, such as heightened ARV resistance, may worsen an already challenging situation.

Infrastructure Problems

Problems with local infrastructure were commonly reported challenges to effective partnerships. Many developing countries have inadequate medical infrastructures and technological capabilities. Communication technology is similarly poor in many low-income nations making consulting and other professional support at long distances difficult to impossible.

One respondent with extensive project planning and implementation experience indicated a need for local skills training particularly at the district level since inadequate planning can jeopardize district as well as local level projects.

High Indigenous Staff Turnover

Several respondents emphasized high rates of indigenous staff and key contact turnover as an obstacle to successful partnering. This can occur for numerous reasons, among them political change, better job opportunities elsewhere, and the impact of the pandemic itself.

Contextual and Cultural Issues

A number of potential challenges arise out of the contexts and cultures in which partnering takes place. Those mentioned or discussed by respondents included the following:

Differences in Medical Culture and "Health Worlds"

In addition to different levels of infrastructure and overall cultural differences, a number of respondents pointed out, directly and indirectly, that partnering organizations can expect to encounter different medical cultures and "health worlds" between developed and developing countries. For example, medical presentations of patients' status in developing countries may be much more abbreviated and less analytical; medical record keeping may be considerably less formal and detailed; the level of deference to professionals may differ between partners; and traditional birth attendants and healers may have a much greater role to play in HIV/AIDS prevention and treatment than some practitioners are accustomed to.

Community Level Depression

The lack of expected local enthusiasm for programs because of chronic community level depression due to HIV/AIDS and its accompanying survival challenges was emphasized by a representative from a major international nongovernmental organization and two other smaller organizations. They believe a multifaceted approach that helps inspire and reinforce hope to community members is needed if such communities are to achieve specific HIV treatment, prevention, and care goals.

Turf Issues

Battles over ownership, responsibility, and control were cited as impediments to effective partnering.

Potential for Personal and Professional Isolation of Volunteers

The risk of isolation was a recognized challenge particularly for volunteers who are deployed without a clearly defined position in the host country and no receiving infrastructure from which they can be oriented to their new environment. This infrastructure might include a community of peers, host-country counterparts, and expatriates.

Volunteer Morale

The prevalence of HIV/AIDS, poor working and living conditions, lack of personal connections, and other frustrations that may arise from international partnering can have a negative impact on the morale of deployed volunteers and the organization as a whole, thus harming the partnering relationship.

SUGGESTED RESPONSES AND SOLUTIONS TO PARTNERING CHALLENGES

Based on responses in the survey, it appears that the challenges outlined above fall into four basic categories. These categories include:

- Realistic expectations
- Organizational responses
- Volunteer placement and support
- Host organization considerations

Realistic Expectations

Results often take longer than expected.

Many respondents suggested that having patience with host and partner organizations and allowing their requirements to set the pace for scaling-up operations will build a stronger relationship in the end.

Programs may cost more than anticipated.

Realistic budgets that provide room for unexpected costs may be better positioned to achieve preset goals. Often, unanticipated extra expenses (such as the need for building physical infrastructure) have been met through private donations.

Plan countermeasures for factors that could slow acceptance of assistance.

This may include actively countering HIV/AIDS based stigmatization, identifying powerful community leaders and community programs that support both the program and have a generally more positive outlook, and enlisting (as many local and internationally partnered organizations have done) traditional and nontraditional educational and entertainment in program activities.

Avoid unrealistic expectations.

A "normal curve" of successful interventions may be the best that can be expected. An organization experienced with operational evaluation of HIV/AIDS projects stated that roughly 25 percent of partnership driven projects fully meet or exceed expectations, 50 percent meet most expectations, and 25 percent fail. Accomplishing project outcomes should therefore not be the only measure of success.

Remain calm and be patient.

A number of respondents emphasized that patience is needed when working with partners particularly with those from economically deprived countries. Attempting to bypass local decision makers or procedures; avoiding sometimes time-consuming meetings and activities; failing to develop local relationships; and failing to identify reliable and effective local counterparts can lead to greater frustration, and ultimately, failure of the project.

Organizational Responses

Encourage equitable long-term relationships.

Partnerships should be based on mutual benefit, respect, shared values, and goals. Those that start small and grow over time have a better chance of maintaining a successful, long-term relationship. This was emphasized by the representative of a university-to-hospital partnership with over 15 years of experience in partnering.

Ensure open communication with partnering organizations, even if it takes more time than expected or planned.

Understand the communication process prior to engaging in a partnership. It may be useful to study and review progress reports from successful partnerships. A number of these successes have been in the field for more

than 15 years and know how to effectively communicate with their partners. They may also have reliable information concerning potential local
counterparts who can be most helpful in maintaining an open dialogue
between partners.

Follow the lead of partner organizations.

Patience and some humility are required for maintaining a successful
long-term relationship. The local partner organization can often teach the
international counterpart about working in its context. Following the local
lead in such situations can build up a reserve of trust and mutual respect
that can be quite useful later on. Experience, evaluation, and reevaluation
are excellent learning tools.

Train counterpart organizations in strategic planning and program evaluation.

Strategic planning and program evaluation are necessary skills for both
short-term success and long-term sustainability of partnerships in local and
international contexts. Continued project growth and support are contin-
gent upon excellent strategies and reliable evaluation.

Volunteer Placement and Support

*Place volunteers in already established programs that are equipped and
experienced in working with the types of volunteers (professions,
numbers, length of stay) expected.*

A number of respondents stated that to work effectively, volunteers
need personal, professional, and administrative support networks. Many
successful volunteer organizations whether secular or faith based, reported
having most of these systems in place.

Survey results also suggested that sending volunteers to un-vetted or
poorly vetted receiving organizations will often create problems. The three
surveyed organizations with higher than average attrition rates acted mostly
as clearinghouses for requesting organizations; focused a large part of their
effort on emergency relief; or expected volunteers to function independently.

*Find local counterparts who are trusted, can break through bureaucratic
logjams, and can act as cultural mediators.*

Linking volunteers with local counterparts can be useful in orienting
them to their new living and working situations. They can provide mediat-
ing services between their in-country colleagues' systems and temporary

personnel (both short and long-term) who might otherwise spend weeks or months trying to accomplish what the counterpart can do in one or two telephone calls. Counterparts can also be helpful in identifying potential and alerting volunteers to potential obstacles to accomplishing their goal.

Because such people are so valuable (and local staff turnover can be high), it is important to insure they remain on-site for considerable periods. If they must leave, they should be involved in identifying and training their successor. As volunteer programs expand or develop new sites, such persons may be helpful in identifying local talent and preexisting networks at these new sites.

Provide experienced volunteer coordinators/supervisors.

Several respondents recommended placing a volunteer coordinator or supervisor in the host country. These people would work in a service similar capacity to the local counterparts. The least expensive way of doing this is to find someone in the receiving organization who is willing and able work on a part time basis and has the appropriate experience. A longer-term volunteer or former volunteer may be appropriate as well.

Host Organization Considerations

Ensure long-term follow through.

It was suggested that long-term follow-through can often be a weakness of local partner organizations—a particularly important consideration in HIV/AIDS related programs. Volunteers should be trained to support their host country counterparts in an effort to maintain a sustained commitment to the program.

Remain committed to the partnership

A number of respondents commented that a resource commitment on the part of the host organization is an important indicator of commitment to a volunteer program. The counterpart organization could provide something in terms of tangible benefits, according to their abilities (i.e., housing) to volunteers as an indication of commitment to the program. Commitment to the partnership could

Balance the cost-benefit value of using volunteers.

Several respondents pointed out the direct costs and opportunity costs of hosting and using volunteers in terms of lost work and resources that could otherwise be used in developing local capacity and sustainability. The danger of fostering dependency on overseas volunteers is also implied in such comments. Therefore, the value of using volunteers (especially short-term people) needs to be balanced against the local opportunity costs (in terms of time and effort expended) of hosting them.

HEALTH CARE PROFESSIONALS: CHALLENGES TO RECRUITING AND RETAINING AN OVERSEAS WORKFORCE

Direct Costs and Opportunity Costs

Volunteers are expensive. For example, it costs roughly $75,000 per year to keep a Peace Corps volunteer in the field. The cost for a midcareer M.D. or Ph.D. may easily be twice that amount when adding other expenses such as a modest salary, family housing costs, home leave, children's education costs, and health insurance.

Ten doctors for 1 year, exclusive of program costs can be budgeted at $1.5 million: 1.25 percent of the annual PEPFAR budget for an average country. Sending one such doctor (including salary) for a 2-week stay to evaluate or consult on existing programs can cost at least $8,000. A 2-week church mission trip to Africa can cost $40,000.

Sustainability

Many organizations prefer to fund and assist in-country organizations and counterparts achieve sustainability on their own, by using in-country personnel and consultants to supplement their own workers, volunteers, and expatriate staff.

Orientation and Staff Time

First time volunteers (except for short-term emergency workers and specialized teams) require orientation, hosting, and support systems. All of this takes time and scarce personnel away from service provision and capacity building. These costs that have to be balanced against the value added by the work and relationship building carried out by volunteers at various levels.

Alternative Sources of Skilled Workers

The United States and other economically advantaged countries are not the only source of skilled workers for developing countries and not always the most appropriate (especially in the case of first time volunteers). Though scarce, a potential supply of skilled staff exist in most countries themselves. Other skilled workers may come from countries where the health culture is closer to that of the host country such as Brazil, Mexico, or India.

Deploying a Proper Mix of Health Professionals

Most of the groups surveyed reported sending short-term doctoral level professionals and nursing volunteers. However, there may be an equal if not greater need for professionals in other areas that support building capacity of the healthcare infrastructure. These might include public health, medical records (particularly important in relation to HIV/AIDS), laboratory and pharmaceutical infrastructure, and human resources management.

Recruitment Challenges

Recruitment of volunteer medical professionals may be difficult, especially for medium and long-term assignments. Early career medical doctors and nurses may have young families and more often than not have large student loan obligations. Midcareer professionals who are willing to interrupt careers and disrupt family life for these assignments can be hard to find. University faculty, for whom such assignments can advance their careers and may be part of their paid professional activities, are a fairly frequent exception. A number of university-based respondents reported having more candidates for these assignments than their programs could accommodate.

Emergency Disasters May Overshadow Chronic Health Conditions

Emergency disasters such as the recent hurricane season in Florida, Hurricane Mitch in 1998, and the Asian Tsunami appear to have taken some of the focus away from the more chronic health problems like the HIV/AIDS pandemic. Although chronic infectious diseases have far-reaching and damaging long-term consequences, they do not appear to have as high status for volunteers and have more complex volunteering requirements.

RECRUITING AND RETAINING OVERSEAS VOLUNTEERS

Volunteer Recruitment Methods

- Most respondents engage in multiple recruitment approaches.
- The Internet is a principal recruiting method, as are returned volunteers and word of mouth (particularly for university based programs).

• University based programs and others cited educational institutions as good sources of volunteer program participants. Universities reported having many more interested faculty than their programs can place.

• Faith-based programs mention faith communities and faith-based organizational networks and news media as good sources. Like university-based programs, they often have more candidates than service options.

Obstacles to Recruitment

When asked to rank the top three challenges to recruitment, respondents placed the following problems highest (in aggregate rank order):

• Volunteer funding
• Length of service (for short and medium as well as long term assignments)
• Family impact and volunteer financial concerns
• Volunteer security

Attrition

In general, reported attrition rates were very low. Twenty-five of the 28 respondents answering this question said attrition was under 10 percent; confined to one or two instances of early departure; or had no attrition at all. Three organizations reported attrition rates of more than 10 percent. One organization places volunteers without consideration to needed skills; one is largely oriented toward quick disaster response missions; and one provided little host country support for volunteers during the high attrition period.

Volunteer Concerns

Principal on-site volunteer concerns were ranked, in aggregate, as follows:

• Feeling isolated
• Health issues
• Safety
• Country politics
• Host culture
• Lack of health infrastructure
• Feeling ineffectual

Combined health and safety concerns far outweigh the other concerns in the list.

FACILITATING IMPROVEMENT IN VOLUNTEER PERFORMANCE

Supportive Context and Larger Networks of Volunteer Support

The most frequently cited assets and resources for good volunteer performance involved various elements of personal, professional and administrative support for their work, both in country and as a part of international health networks. Specific aspects of these conditions that facilitated volunteer performance include:

- Existence of personal and professional support systems
- Trusted and resourceful local counterparts
- Opportunities to learn from locals
- Long term presence of U.S. organization in country with good local relationships
- Well-defined volunteer responsibilities (especially for short-term volunteers)
- Good peer support and relationships (especially for doctors)
- Basic needs met

CROSS-CULTURAL TRAINING

Culture, Language, Medical Culture, and Health Worlds

The issues of culture shock and culture clash as noted earlier, are particularly complex when dealing with the HIV/AIDS pandemic. Respondents indicated there are several levels to these issues, some of which can be ameliorated through training. As Table D-2 indicates, a majority of respondents provide and recommend some form of U.S.-based cultural training prior to in-country placement. This can range from provision of a manual to the 7-month U.S. and in-country culture and language program required by 3-year volunteers. Organizations that do not provide U.S.-based cultural training often emphasize in-country cultural training. Some organizations refuse applicants with no significant experience living and working in cultures other than their own.

It appears that most organizations do not spend much time discussing differences in medical cultures or indigenous languages. Even when English is the working language, it can be nuanced very differently in another country creating communication barriers.

TABLE D-2 Cross-Cultural Training

Cultural Training Methods	Provides Training	Training Manual	Training Video	1-Day Course	2–14-Day Course	Longer Course	In-Country Training	Minimal or Informal
No. of Responding Organizations Using Method	24	13	5	5	8	4	12	7

SUMMARY

In summary, volunteers seem to function best when peer support, opportunities for positive interaction with locals and expatriates, and resources for personal, professional, and bureaucratic problem solving are in place.

These responses support observations drawn from discussions of attrition and organizational partnering that point to the successes of well-established partnerships with well defined roles and good supervision as the best contexts for effective volunteer performance. They also suggest that volunteer performance and achievement of objectives are enhanced when health networks have solid and mutually reinforcing relationships at all levels: local, in-country, regional, and international. In this way, local health cultures can be respected and their resources employed to full advantage (for example in organizing traditional birth attendants to support voluntary counseling, testing, and prevention of mother-to-child transmission and in combining HIV work with broader health and development goals). At the same time, volunteers, other expatriate health professionals, and their local counterparts and colleagues can fully utilize resources such as distance learning, international, consulting and sources of information, capacity building, and supply that can be made available through international partnering.

Appendix E

E-Health and the HIV/AIDS Epidemic: Using Technology to Support U.S. Workforce Expansion and Local Capacity Building in PEPFAR Nations

Holly Ladd and Rebecca Riccio

SATELLIFE

SUMMARY

The vast scope of the HIV/AIDS pandemic has generated an unprecedented need for medical services in low-resource countries, taxing already over-burdened and understaffed health care systems. As the World Health Organization (WHO) reported at a 2002 joint meeting with the World Bank in Addis Ababa:

> There is an emerging crisis of health manpower in Africa. The situation threatens to defeat the efforts of African governments, private health care providers, NGOs, and donors for health improvement. Training programmes unsuited to changing health conditions, inadequate cooperation among the many parties concerned, and the losses of staff to opportunities outside Africa risk making Africa's health care facilities barely able to function for lack of qualified, motivated doctors, nurses and other health workers. This situation is made even worse by the AIDS epidemic, which reduces further the availability of trained health workers by staff deaths and increases the demand for health care.[1]

To address the urgent need for more health workers, the President's Emergency Plan for AIDS Relief (PEPFAR) calls for the placement of U.S.

---

[1]WHO Report at Building Strategic Partnerships in Education and Health, a WHO/World Bank Meeting, Addis Ababa, January 2002, as reported by Ntiro, Simba, et al. in Information and Communication Technologies and Continuing Medical Education in East and Southern Africa, Report of a Conference held in Moshi Tanzania, 8–10 April 2003, Research Report 17, June 2003. http://www.ftpiicd.org/files/research/reports/report17.pdf.

medical volunteers to complement and augment the capacity of local health workers in PEPFAR countries.[2] The PEPFAR further identifies telemedicine as a tool to support these efforts.[3] The experience of multiple organizations with experience in telemedicine, or more broadly defined, e-health, in low-resource countries has shown that while technology might be used to extend the presence of United States medical volunteers and build the capacity of local health professionals to combat HIV/AIDS, expectations about what they can achieve must be informed by a realistic understanding of the limited infrastructure and skills available to support them on the ground. Moreover, a commitment to using e-health should be driven by identified, real demands for improved access to information, data, training, etc., to combat HIV/AIDS and an understanding of how technology can meet those demands, rather than by a perception of e-health as an end unto itself. The most cost-effective and successful interventions are likely to be those that creatively leverage existing infrastructure and skills, such as low bandwidth e-mail, or those that introduce new technologies that are relatively inexpensive and easily adoptable, such as handheld computers and cellular telephones. A variety of e-health projects that follow these guidelines are already in existence and should be evaluated and considered as possible resource partners for a United States volunteer program before new projects are initiated.

BACKGROUND:
HEALTH SYSTEMS CAPACITY IN PEPFAR COUNTRIES

Those countries hit hardest by HIV/AIDS face acute shortages of trained medical personnel. As Table E-1 indicates, the availability of physicians, nurses, and midwives per 100,000 people is limited in all 15 PEFAR countries.

The availability of health care in these countries can be expanded in many ways, including:

1. Recruiting and training new health workers (all cadres) from the local population.

2. Expanding the capacity of the existing local workforce by, for example, upgrading skills or expanding health workers' reach into underserved areas.

---

[2]The President's Emergency Plan for AIDS Relief, p. 37.
[3]PEPFAR, p. 37.

TABLE E-1 Nurses, Midwives, and Physicians per 100,000 Population

15 PEPFAR Focus Countries	Nurses and Midwives per 100,000 Population	Physicians per 100,000 Population
Botswana	241.0785	28.7644
Côte d'Ivoire	46.2024	9
Ethiopia	20.5333	2.8581
Guyana	229	48.2
Haiti	10.7	25
Kenya	90.1	13.2
Mozambique	28.4303	2.4354
Namibia	284	29.5
Nigeria	118.5	26.916
Rwanda	21.0941	1.8737
South Africa	388.01	69.2095
Tanzania	36.6409	2.2659
Uganda	8.8	4.7
Viet Nam	74.752	53.4455
Zambia	113.1	6.9

SOURCE: World Health Organization, *Global Atlas,* last updated 26/Oct/04.

3. Increasing the number of foreign national health professionals working in PEPFAR countries, including U.S. medical volunteers.

4. Adding support for ancillary and administrative tasks to relieve health workers' time for more patient care.

5. Reorganizing health care delivery to realize more efficiency.

These approaches are compatible with the PEPFAR's strategy for "rapidly training and mobilizing health care personnel to provide treatment services."[4] To facilitate this effort, the PEPFAR explicitly states that "telemedicine and distance education can be used to build the skills of health professionals in the focus countries and strengthen local, national, and international connections among medical institutions."[5]

WHAT IS E-HEALTH?

A variety of technologies—and terms to describe their use—have been developed to facilitate the delivery of health care over long distances

---

[4]PEPFAR, pp. 36–37.
[5]PEPFAR, p. 37.

throughout the world. "Telemedicine" implies the use of technology to support the delivery of clinical services, such as telesurgery or teleradiology. "Telehealth" is sometimes used synonymously, but often connotes the use of technology in health-related communication and information exchange, including distance training. "Information and communication technology (ICT) for health" can overlap with both of these concepts, but is also used to describe the use of technology to realize time and cost efficiencies and quality improvement in day-to-day practice, such as the use of handheld computers for routine data collection.

The World Health Organization has adopted the use of the term "e-health" to encompass the whole range of technologies and applications that have variously been identified as telemedicine, telehealth, and ICT for health, and advocates their use to improve health care delivery in a variety of circumstances.[6] Throughout this paper, the term "e-health" will refer broadly to the exchange of actionable information over distance to facilitate both health service delivery and capacity building within the health sector.

The successful adoption of e-health in both low-resource and industrialized countries has enabled health professionals to overcome time and distance barriers and bring their expertise to poor and isolated communities that might otherwise be denied basic health services. Solutions need not be complicated or expensive to be effective. Even relatively simple technology such as e-mail can, for example, enable a United States health worker stationed in a capital city to communicate with local counterparts in rural villages about HIV/AIDS-related skin conditions, or enable peers separated by vast distances to communicate and consult. Simple e-mail-based discussion groups have proven to be an excellent forum for south-to-south support, knowledge building and sharing, and informal training within the global health community, as evidenced by SATELLIFE's electronic discussion groups AFRO-NETS and E-Drug. The dissemination of medical literature via e-mail in electronic publications such as *HealthNet News* and *HealthNet News AIDS* is both cost-effective and responsive to real needs.[7]

E-health also opens up a wide range of training and continuing medical education opportunities. Several institutions have successfully implemented distance training and continuing medical education programs, enabling a

---

[6]*E-Health*, Report by the Secretariat, WHO, December 2004. See also, *A Health Telematics Policy in Support of WHO's Health-for-All Strategy for Global Health Development*, Report on the WHO Group Consultation on Health Telematics, 11–16 December, Geneva, 1997; WHO, 1998, available at http://whqlibdoc.who.int/hq/1998/WHO_DGO_98.1.pdf.

[7]See the SATELLIFE website, http://www.healthnet.org.

Focus on South Africa: Cell Life

More than 90 percent of South Africa is covered by cellular networks, and more than a third of all South Africans currently use cell phones. Cell-Life supports home-based care providers who collect medical and socio-economic data from patients through the use of applications on their cellular phones. Data are relayed over a GSM network to the central database. Medical and administrative staff access the data via a secure Internet connection for analysis. Communication and feedback are also provided to home-based care providers via SMS text messaging.

SOURCE: http://www.cell-life2.os.org.za/home/home.html.

small pool of educators to reach a wider audience than would otherwise be possible and to extend education and training into areas where it would otherwise be unavailable.[8] A comprehensive and insightful analysis of the use of ICT to support continuing medical education emerged from a 2003 joint meeting sponsored the Centre for Educational Development in Health (CEDHA; Arusha, Tanzania), the Institute for International Communications Development (IICD; the Netherlands), and CORDAID (the Netherlands). The meeting report examines the constraints and opportunities for CME presented by ICT and outlines steps for moving forward in Uganda, Tanzania, Zambia, and Kenya.[9]

E-health has been practiced long enough for valuable lessons learned and best practices to have emerged. Some of the earliest e-health projects were sponsored by the International Telecommunications Union, which has since documented its lessons learned.[10] Reproductive Health Outlook, the reproductive health website produced by Program for Appropriate Technology in Health (PATH), has produced a comprehensive analysis of the use of ICT for health in low-resource settings.[11] The Telemedicine Information Exchange hosts a database of international and U.S.-based telemedicine

---

[8]Kwankam, S. Yukap. October 2004. What e-Health can offer, *Bulletin of the World Health Organization.*82(10):800–801.

[9]This report is available at http://www.ftpiicd.org/files/research/reports/report17.pdf.

[10]This report is available at http://www2.telemed.no/publikasjoner/nedlastbare/telecomm_dev_bureau%20.doc.

[11]This report is available at http://www.rho.org/html/ict.htm.

projects and contains useful references about a wide range of related issues.[12]

THE TECHNOLOGY BEHIND E-HEALTH

Pipeline Technologies

An assessment of the potential to utilize e-health in any environment must first take into consideration the "pipeline" technologies that might be used. These are the networking mechanisms that convey information and data from one point to another. Their availability and cost vary considerably from country to country, and even within country, and so must be assessed on a case-by-case basis. Other factors that must be considered in assessing pipeline technologies include speed, capacity (bandwidth or volume), and cost.

Access to these technologies varies along a continuum: in urban areas, high bandwidth access is usually available to medical and teaching institutions, while in rural areas, only radios or cellular telephones may be available. The availability of these technologies is determined primarily by national telecom policy and market forces, so organizations contemplating the introduction of e-health under time and financial constraints are well-advised to work within the range of the continuum available in their targeted environment.

Table E-2 offers a list of the most widely used pipeline technologies in low-resource environments, as well as the types of hardware and software associated with using them.

CONSTRAINTS TO USING E-HEALTH

Limitations of Technology

While all of the technologies described above are being used to varying degrees in low-resource countries, including those covered by PEPFAR, there are significant limitations that must be considered in planning e-health projects. Conditions that preclude the use of certain types of technologies in some environments include:

1. Inadequate (sometimes nonexistent) telecommunication infrastructure and power supply to support networking beyond urban areas

---

[12]See the Telemedicine Information Exchange web site, http://tie.telemed.org.

TABLE E-2 Technologies and Related Tools Associated with E-Health in Low-Resource Environments

Distribution/ Connectivity	Local Networking	Software Hardware	Applications[a]
Satellites	LAN	Satellite ground	Basic office packages
DSL/Broadband	WAN–VSAT	station	Accounting
Continuous data feed	Wi-Fi	Server/	Database
Continuous radio feed	Local Internet	Networking	Communications
VSAT	service	hardware	Electronic medical
Dial-up	"Sneaker"	(router, hub	record
Landline/Modem	network	etc.)	Reference texts
Cell (GSM modem)	(motorbike,	Computer	
Radio (two-way)	bicycle, and	workstations	
Radio (broadcast)	feet)	Laptop	
		Handheld computer	
		Cell phone	
		Pager	
		Smart card reader	
		Scanner	
		GPS	
		Landline phone	
		Digital camera	
		Pencil and paper	

[a]The choice of appropriate software will be driven both by function and by the hardware available, yielding a range of options too broad to address in this paper. As the conceptualization of e-health projects to support United States medical volunteers under PEPFAR evolves and the number of variables is reduced, the range of appropriate software will become increasingly evident.

2. Inadequate resources for institutions and facilities to acquire and sustain the ongoing use of technology

3. Lack of local skills to use the technology, both among the technologists who need to support e-health systems and among the health professionals who will use them

Any one or more of these factors can inhibit health workers' access to the benefits of e-health. For example, a recent study done to determine the feasibility of expanding African universities' access to scientific literature provided the following data on the cost—frequently prohibitive—of electronic access (see Table E-3).

These conditions do not prelude the use of e-health, but they do dictate which types of technology are most appropriate in certain environments. The designers of e-health projects are well-advised to find creative technol-

TABLE E-3 Comparative Bandwidth Costs: United States, Uganda, and Nigeria

Country	Institution	Current bandwidth (downlink/uplink)	Cost/month	Cost per kbps per month
United States	n/a	1.5 Mbps	US$399	$0.266
Uganda	Makerere University	1500 Kbps/ 786 kbps	US$22,500	$9.84
Nigeria	Obafemi Awolowo University	512 Kbps/ 128 kbps	US$12,800	$20.00

SOURCE: IDRC. Open and Closed Skies: Satellite Access in Africa, the International Development Research Centre (IDRC), Canada, 2004. This report is available at http://web.idrc.ca/en/ev-51227-201-1-DO_TOPIC.html.

ogy solutions within these constraints rather than to invest the time and resources that would be required to change the technology environment. Experience has shown that when the introduction of technology is compatible with existing infrastructure and skills, it is possible to achieve sustainable, cost-effective results.

Limitations of Current Practice

Current practice, clinical and administrative, may not be easily adaptable to e-health. E-health is a tool to complement health care services; it cannot correct weaknesses or problems within health care systems or function well in environments characterized by:

1, Poor data-management practices or health information systems (HIS)
2. Obstructionist politics around information "ownership"
3. Lack of leadership or vision
4. Other political, systemic, or institutional barriers, such as staff resistance to technology

Limitations of the Existing Workforce

The use of e-health to extend the United States workforce presence will require the cooperation of and coordination with the existing local workforce, which, as has been discussed, is already overburdened by enormous

---

Focus on Haiti: Partners in Health, Zanmi Lasante

Health workers at Zanmi Lasante in Cange, Haiti consult with counterparts at Partners in Health in Boston, Massachusetts using desktop computers and a satellite connection to share web-based records for clinical management. The system allows patient consultation and care decisions to be made remotely.

SOURCE: www.pih.org.

---

caseloads, reporting requirements, training and supervision, etc. E-health interventions must be perceived as collaborative and constructive, resulting in visible benefits rather than increasing the workload, if they are to receive the local support they need to succeed.

E-Health in Action: The Uganda Health Information Network

Experience has shown that projects that recognize and work within these constraints can be very successful. Working in partnership with Uganda Chartered HealthNet (UCH), SATELLIFE has created the Uganda Health Information Network (UHIN) to support health data and information exchange. The network combines the use of handheld computers (also known as personal digital assistants or PDAs), the local GSM cellular telephone network, and self-contained relay stations or "Jacks," to provide a two-way flow of data and information between health facilities in Mbale and Rakai Districts and the Ministry of Health in Kampala. Now moving into its second year of operation, UHIN is independently owned and man-

---

**Focus on South Africa: Africa Centre for
Health and Populations Studies**

An "HIV Confidant" carries confidential HIV test results to remote locations on handheld computers (PDAs) customized by the Africa Centre. The device features confidential double-key entry for both provider and patient, records patient consent, and tracks requests for results.

SOURCE: http://www.africacentre.org.za

aged by UCH, an independent NGO based at Makerere University Faculty of Medicine. Two routine data collection forms have been converted to the PDA format, enabling health facilities in the target districts to submit their monthly data reports to the Ministry of Health via the network. A cost-effectiveness study has shown that UHIN results in a 25 percent cost savings in this routine data collection, a figure that the project partners expect to increase as additional data collection forms are converted to the PDA. The network has resulted in significant local capacity building, both at UCH, which has acquired the technical and administrative skills to manage the network, and at the networked facilities in Mbale and Rakai, which are not only improving their data collection capacity but also receiving valuable content through the network.[13]

E-HEALTH AND HIV/AIDS

Understanding the Environment, Identifying Real Demands

The design of e-health programs to expand the United States workforce and build local capacity in PEPFAR countries must complement the existing in-country networks of HIV/AIDS care providers. Decentralization has resulted in an expansion of the network of health workers engaged in HIV/AIDS, ranging from highly trained, hospital-based medical staff in urban settings to community volunteers in rural villages. A U.S. volunteer can theoretically be located anywhere and/or communicate with anyone within the network of hospitals, clinics, research and academic institutions, hospices, voluntary counseling and treatment (VCT) centers, orphan and vulnerable children (OVC)-focused organizations, counseling and support groups, home-based care, education and training programs, and work-based centers. UNAIDS has suggested that ICT can be effective in supporting this network all the way down to the community level,[14] but several questions must be answered, such as: Where will volunteers be placed? With whom will they communicate? About what? And why?

Answering these questions may prove far more complicated than might be expected, as illustrated by an examination of record keeping needs related to anti-retroviral drugs (ARV), an area in which e-health would seem to be a natural solution. The widespread use of ARV in developing coun-

---

[13]See the UHIN website at http://www.pda.healthnet.org.

[14]Potential for ICT to Support Community Health Organizations, 2004 UNAIDS Report on the Global AIDS Epidemic, Section 2. This report is available at http://www.unaids.org/bangkok2004/GAR2004_html/GAR2004_00_en.htm.

tries requires record keeping at both the patient and facility level, yet the practice and quality of record keeping varies widely between and within countries. Medical records are not standardized within or across PEPFAR countries. Local health clinics may not keep patient records and instead may rely on the care provider and the patients to remember the illness and treatments previously prescribed. In some cases patients carry a "record" with them that includes dates of visits and health workers' hand written notes. Each time patients visit a health provider, they must bring the record with them. Few, if any, rural clinics maintain electronic records for either patient care or clinic utilization. Rather, information is recorded as a tick mark in a ledger. The entries are counted at the end of the month and copied over onto paper reporting forms that are collected or sent on to the next higher level of care to be aggregated into regional and national level reports.

Another important consideration is that each clinic must fill out multiple, often duplicative reports, the number and nature of which is determined by the number of vertically funded programs (and donors) they are drawing resources from. These reporting requirements, while perhaps important for a range of needs, nevertheless diminish the amount time a care provider has for direct patient care.

Multiple discussions are underway in an attempt to agree upon a uniform data set across all ARV programs, but many organizations have developed their own EMR or database, reflecting a desire to continue using their own product. At the same time several projects are underway to introduce clinic level patient record keeping using computers, handheld computers and smart cards. These activities, sometimes complementary, sometimes mutually exclusive, illustrate that while the tools of e-health can be used to meet the record keeping and data collection demands generated by the widespread use of ARV, they can only be maximally effective only if the underlying organizational, logistical, and political issues are addressed, and efforts are coordinated at multiple levels.[15]

Targeted Content, Appropriate Technology

Understanding the environment in which volunteers will be placed, both to maximize the impact of their presence in country and to facilitate

---

[15]Though it is beyond the scope of this paper to explore issues regarding volunteer selection and placement in detail, this illustration also suggests that the range of expertise required is not limited to physicians and nurses, but may also include nonclinical expertise in systems management, information technology, records, pharmaceuticals, palliative care, work flow management, etc.

Focus on Rwanda: Central Hospital, Kigali— Institute of Tropical Medicine, Antwerp

An on-site training course on the use of ARV is conducted at the Central Hospital by ITM staff, then followed up by remote e-mail support, continuing training, and access to a community of practice that reinforces the theoretical course.

SOURCE: http://telemedicine.itg.be/telemedicine/site/Default.asp?WPID=59.

---

their ability to build local work force capacity, makes it possible then to consider how e-health can facilitate their work, and the content they will need to exchange with their local counterparts. Virtually any two points within the network of HIV/AIDS caregivers can be linked, and the content they exchange can range from simple e-mail messages and data files to full-color images and streaming video, but not all solutions are viable or cost-effective. Key issues to consider in selecting which technology is the most appropriate include: How often will they need to be in touch? How critical is it that they have access to each other on demand? What volume of information will they be exchanging? Will it be a one-way flow or a two-way flow? How many other people may need to see the information? Will they be exchanging confidential information?

The answers to these questions, paired with an understanding of the IT environment, make it possible to design appropriate e-health programs. The range of options is illustrated in Table E-4.

Personal Digital Assistants (PDAs) and HIV/AIDS

SATELLIFE has found that PDAs lend themselves especially well to information dissemination and data collection and analysis. Together with the WHO, SATELLIFE is testing the use of PDAs to keep facility-level patient ARV care records (an "ARV patient card"), tracking cohorts of patients on ARV and their status. SATELLIFE's longer-term goal is to develop an "HIV/AIDS PDA" that combines many of the PDA applications that SATELLIFE has already successfully tested, but is specifically targeted toward the needs of HIV/AIDS caregivers. Its functions would include the following.

1. *Patient screening and rapid assessment.* For example, a local nurse can interview patients using an interactive PDA form, receive a recommendation, and triage patients for a physician.

TABLE E-4 E-Health Options

Networking Technologies Available	E-Health Applications Possible
Broadband Internet (via satellite, telephone)	Web-based information sharing, live teleconferencing
Low bandwidth e-mail	Consulting, program coordination, routine communication, text only journals, discussion groups, and other references
Cell phone	Consulting, program coordination, routine communication, patient reminders, simple data reporting
Multiple technologies (including handhelds, smart phones)	Patient record exchange, training and CME, reporting, supervisory support, inventory management, secondary diagnosis, text and reference material, e-books, data collection and reporting, databases, voice recording, digital photos, etc.

2. *Preliminary diagnosis.* For example, a nurse can use an interactive PDA form to determine whether a patient should be tested for HIV/AIDS, without that person needing to see a physician.

3. *ARV management.* For example, a community health volunteer can use a PDA to keep track of ARV regimens to support compliance during household visits.

4. *Patient records, patient tracking.* For example, each patient can be issued a smart card containing his or her personal record which can be updated on the PDA at each visit. In the case of orphans, vital documents, identification, photos, etc., could also be recorded to facilitate care-giving and preserve vital records in the absence of family support mechanisms.

5. *Data collection, including demographic surveys.* Virtually any data that is routinely collected using pencil and paper can be translated into an electronic form. (Open-ended questions are less adaptable to this format.)

6. *Information dissemination and knowledge building.* PDAs can hold a virtual library of resources, including treatment guidelines, medical references and text books, etc.

COST EFFECTIVENESS OF E-HEALTH

Documented evidence regarding the cost effectiveness of e-health interventions overall, including in industrialized countries, is limited, although this reflects a lack of study, rather than a lack of cost-savings.[16] However, there is some evidence that low-bandwidth technology can be especially cost effective in resource poor countries.[17]

The cost effectiveness study by SATELLIFE and Uganda Chartered HealthNet is one of the few rigorous studies available on the cost effectiveness of handheld computers, indicating a 25 percent savings in the cost of data collection as opposed to paper and pencil methods.[18] Other partners with whom SATELLIFE has worked to establish PDA capacity, including the American Red Cross, the Uganda Red Cross, and Management Sciences for Health, have not conducted comprehensive studies, but have reported significant cost savings to SATELLIFE based on standard project evaluations.[19]

The long-term sustainability of a project must factor into considerations of cost effectiveness. Short-term analysis may reflect savings that can quickly be lost if the host institution is encumbered with an unsustainable program once donor funding is exhausted. Therefore, the design of e-health programs must account for the ongoing costs of training, hardware and software maintenance, connectivity (Internet, telephone), and other recurring expenses.

E-HEALTH, HIV/AIDS, AND VOLUNTEERS

E-health can factor into the design of a program for United States medical volunteers working in or with PEPFAR countries in a variety of ways. The extent and nature of an e-health component in the volunteer program will depend on how the program itself is ultimately designed, but several models should be considered:

---

[16]Systematic review of cost effectiveness studies of telemedicine interventions. BMJ 2002; 324:1434-1437, available at http://bmj.bmjjournals.com/cgi/content/full/324/7351/1434; Kwankam, S. Yunkap, Bulletin of the WHO, pp. 800–801.

[17]Frasier and McGrath, Information technology and telemedicine in sub-Saharan Africa. *BMJ.* 2000. 321(7259):465-466, available at http://bmj.bmjjournals.com/cgi/content/full/321/7259/465).

[18]This study is available at http://www.healthnet.org/coststudy.php.

[19]Presentations on two of these projects were made at Handheld Computers in Africa: Exploring the Promise for the Health Sector, a conference sponsored by SATELLIFE, Uganda Chartered HealthNet and IDRC, May 12–13, 2004, Entebbe, Uganda. For more information on the Uganda Red Cross project, see http://pda.healthnet.org/docs/fredrick_urcs_presentation. ppt. For more information on the MSH project, see http://pda.healthnet.org/docs/ arin_conf_presentation.pp.

Focus on Uganda:
Satellife, Uganda Chartered HealthNet, Makerere University

The Uganda Health Information Network enables health workers in Mbale and Rakai districts to use handheld computers (PDAs) to collect data, receive training and reference materials, and send and receive e-mail. Users connect to the network using the infrared beam of their PDAs to connect or "hot sync" with an access device which in turn communicates with a central server in Kampala via the GSM cellular network. The network facilitates both routine data collection and reporting between rural health facilities and the District Health Offices and continuing medical education.

SOURCE: http://www.pda.healthnet.org.

E-Health to Support Volunteers

A variety of volunteer placement programs are already utilizing tools associated with e-health to support overseas assignments, and can serve as models for the proposed PEPFAR volunteer initiative. For example, St. George's Hospital in London uses an e-mail health consultation service for overseas volunteers, who use the system to address diverse medical concerns and receive collegial support.[20] Programs such as the Peace Corps are also likely to have useful models that could be adapted.

E-Health to Extend the Reach of Volunteers into Remote Areas

Several models exist in which e-health is used to extend the reach of specialized services into rural areas or to build local capacity. For example, Dr. Roy Colven of the University of Washington, working in partnership with the MRC Telemedicine Research Council, has established a teledermatology project at the University of Cape Town in South Africa. The network will serve regions of southern Africa that have limited access to health care providers. Using e-mail and digital cameras, remote practitioners send photographs of HIV/AIDS-related skin disorders to consulting physicians working in Cape Town, who review the digital images for consultation and diagnosis.[21]

---

[20]E-mail consultations in international health. *Lancet* 2000; 356(9224):138.

[21]For more information on this project, see http://archives.thedaily.washington.edu/search.lasso?-database=DailyWebSQL&-table=Articles&-response=searchpage.lasso&-keyField=__Record_ID__&-keyValue=9983&-search).

Also in South Africa, the Tsilitwa telehealth project enables nurses to use a web camera to send live pictures of a patient over a wireless network to a doctor at the University of Cape Town. Simultaneously, they can consult live via telephone about the patient. Tsilitwa is an extremely poor and remote village that is difficult to reach by public transportation and has virtually no other means of communication beyond this network.[22]

E-Health to Provide Remote Support and to
Facilitate Institutional Relationships

One model for the effective engagement of volunteers may include an on-site visit and "rotation" by a senior level health provider (defined as a care provider at a peer level who has had significant HIV/AIDS care and treatment or patient management experience in their own practice) who is able to establish a trusting peer relationship with a provider or care site in a PEPFAR country and makes a commitment to maintain a relationship with that provider or clinic. This relationship can continue after the volunteer returns home through "e-twinning," the use of e-health tools to provide:

- Sustained communication and consultations
- Access to reference and resource materials not available in the PEPFAR country
- Regular updates of relevant medical and clinical information
- A peer network (e.g., e-mail discussion groups) that enables the volunteer and the PEPFAR country program to call upon the resources of a community of practice

Building on Existing Programs

As an e-health component of the United States volunteer program is developed, it will be important to assess and, where possible, leverage existing programs. Formal e-health strategies have been adopted by several PEPFAR countries, both at the national and institutional level. Examples include:

- The Zambian Ministry of Health has been actively working to

---

[22]The South African NGO Bridges.org has prepared a case study on this project, available at http://www.bridges.org/iicd_casestudies/tsilitwa_telehealth/.

Focus on Mozambique : Empresa Nacional de Telecomunicações de Moçambique (TDM), Maputo and Beira Central Hospitals, WDS Technologies of Switzerland

Medical personnel at central hospitals in Maputo and Beira engage in teleconsultation and teleradiology using a terrestrial and satellite links to exchange histories, images, and test results.

SOURCE: http://www2.telemed.no/publikasjoner/nedlastbare/telecomm_dev_bureau%20.doc.

develop a national telehealth strategy as a means of extending health services throughout the country.[23]

• In Tanzania, the Muhimbili University Health Exchange Forum has been established "to facilitate communication and the flow of health information between healthworkers in the districts and regions of Tanzania and health experts and postgraduate students of Muhimbili."[24]

• In Uganda, the Academic Alliance for AIDS Care and Prevention in Africa has identified telemedicine as one of the tools it will use to support the training efforts at the Infectious Disease Institute in Kampala.[25]

• South Africa has a national telehealth strategy that includes hospitals and universities, with the goal "to make telemedicine live up to its potential as a valuable tool to improve access to high quality and cost effective health care services in South Africa."[26]

Existing federally-funded programs such as the Global HIV/AIDS Program, Office for the Advancement of Telehealth, at the U.S. Department of Health and Human Services, should also be explored for possible linkages, models, and lessons learned.[27]

---

[23]Chanda, Kenneth, Outline of telehealth development in Zambia, 1 September 2004, http://209.250.143.167/atp/_disc1/00000018.htm.

[24]The Muhimbili Health Exchange Forum website is http://www.muhef.or.tz/.

[25]The website on the training program of the Academic Alliance for AIDS Care and Prevention in Africa is http://www.aaacp.org/training.index.html.

[26]This report is available at http://www.kznhealth.gov.za/telemedicine1.pdf.

[27]The website for the HRSA Global HIV/AIDS Program is http://hab.hrsa.gov/special/global.htm.

KEY CONSIDERATIONS

Over the course of its 16 years in implementing e-health projects throughout Africa, Asia, and Latin America, SATELLIFE has learned that a variety of considerations beyond content and technology must factor into the design of a successful program. These lessons include the following.

• Technology is disruptive. E-health programs have the potential to upset existing hierarchies and work patterns and procedures, creating both political and administrative conflicts. Change management must be deliberate and cautious.

• Information ownership is a politically charged issue. Control of information and data is heavily tied to power relationships at many levels. E-health programs must be sensitive to the politics and relationships in place from the Ministry of Health to the front-line community volunteer.

• Technology is a tool, not a solution. E-health in and of itself cannot fix health systems, nor is it a substitute for good practices. Existing practices must be understood and factored into the design of e-health programs.

• Back-up, security, and privacy issues should be considered early in the design process. Systems must be designed with redundancy and security, and protocols must be established to maintain them from the outset. The level of privacy and confidentiality required for information and data exchange must be understood before the technology and software are selected. They must be built into the system.

• Explore alternative power sources (battery, solar, generator). Creative solutions for supplying power may extend the reach of some technologies into rural areas.

• E-health programs should not create additional burdens for health workers if the technology is to be adopted successfully. E-health programs must be seen as part of the solution, not part of the problem, and must be inclusive and collaborative.

• A local champion can ensure the success of a project. It is imperative to find local advocates who know the system, are invested in e-health, and are invested to influence key stakeholders.

• Training of end users and technologists must be thorough, and ongoing support must be available until the technology is fully adopted. Training of trainers is essential to ensure that second-generation users will be successful.

• The long-term sustainability of the project must be considered from the beginning—not when funding is winding down—so that local partners are not encumbered with unmanageable recurring expenses.

• Many local models of successful e-health programs already exist.

Partnering with these programs can be far more cost-effective and responsive to local needs than launching new projects.

CONCLUSION

E-health has proven to be a cost-effective mechanism for enabling health workers to overcome barriers of time and distance and to exchange actionable information and data relating to health service delivery in multiple settings in low-resource environments. Successful projects are demand-driven and remain responsive to both local content needs and existing practices. They are also grounded within the range of the technology "continuum" that is realistically available to them, creatively adopting applications that are compatible with the local telecommunications infrastructure.

Within the context of a United States medical volunteer program, e-health has the potential to provide support to volunteers, to extend the reach of volunteers into remote areas, and to serve as a conduit for capacity building and support between volunteers and local counterparts. Sufficient functional models exist to merit a more comprehensive inventory of e-health activities in each PEPFAR country to determine whether the placement of volunteers may be able to leverage existing initiatives, although such a determination should be made within the perspective of other urgent critical needs.

Appendix F

ICT Considerations to Support PEPFAR Activities

Ronaldo Lima, M.Sc.
International AIDS Vaccine Initiative

GENERAL CONSIDERATIONS TOWARD IMPLEMENTING ICT IN DEVELOPING COUNTRIES

Information and communication technologies (ICTs) are critical to evaluate and analyze clinical information, as well as to improve general access to information. ICTs also hold great potential for narrowing the information gap faced by health care professionals. Health professionals not only can read many of the latest medical journals on-line, but they can also communicate directly with other professionals from anywhere in the world (Storey, 1999). Access to electronic libraries and specialized databases, phone and e-mail communication, discussion groups, video and web conference, and distance learning are some examples of what ICT tools can provide. Thus, ICTs offer potentially powerful tools to improve health, contribute to poverty elimination and speed up the process of human development.

What Is an ICT?

ICTs include a broad spectrum of communication technologies from radio, film, television, press, telephone, and Internet to more participatory forms such as theater, video, or storytelling. "New" ICTs tend to focus on the electronic or digital end of the spectrum such as e-mail, the Internet, mobile phones, and digital (video) cameras (Chetley, 2001).

Important Key Points to Consider:

1. Communication, not technology, should be the central concern.
2. Strong health systems and other basic services are essential for effective use of ICTs.
3. Increased capacity to access, organize, repackage, and use information effectively is a major priority.
4. Local ownership, participation, and content improve the relevance of ICT activities.
5. ICTs should complement other communication work and be integrated into broader programs.

It is useful to distinguish between the parts of information and communication technology by looking at the:

* technology itself,
* information that the technology helps to convey, and
* communication process that the technology is meant to facilitate and through which the information is meant to flow.

An issue that has been discussed in the past few years and is also a factor that drives the technological push is the concept of a "digital divide." The G-8 Digital Opportunity Taskforce (DOT Force) defines it as "unequal possibilities to access and contribute to information, knowledge, and networks as well as to benefit from the development enhancing capabilities of ICT"(Chetley, 2001).

The digital divide is an integral part of a much broader and more intractable "development divide." The likelihood that people in low-income countries can improve their life chances is often sharply limited not only by their lack of access to modern means of communication and sources of information, but also by a complex network of constraints ranging from unresolved problems of poverty and injustice in their own societies (Alcantara, 2001).

To a very large degree, low-income countries depend on foreign institutions and actors to create both an adequate telecommunications infrastructure and a regulatory framework that is progressive and fair. Development assistance is crucial in this regard. The effort is likely to be more effective if it takes place within the context of national ICT strategies, which make explicit the need to adapt available technical and economic options to the needs of specific countries. These strategies should also provide a framework for better national coordination of many disparate efforts, by NGOs and others, to use ICTs to improve public administration and social services, and to support democracy in developing countries (Alcantara, 2001).

However, few projects monitor and evaluate ICT outcomes, especially local impact. Where ICT evaluation has been carried out, for example with telecentres in Latin America and the Caribbean, results tend to be used by external donors, rather than by the people involved (Chetley, 2001; Delgadillo and Borja, 1999).

The Economic Commission for Africa describes health-related ICT approaches in Africa as "islands of donor-supported projects that have little impact on the growing health crisis because they often prove too costly to be replicable." It says an African-driven approach could lead to more appropriate interventions to meet the continent's needs (Chetley, 2001).

Some lessons can be drawn about how to increase the relevance of ICTs as tools for better health and development. These include the need to (Chetley, 2001):

- strengthen and build upon basic systems and infrastructure;
- invest heavily in strengthening local human resources and capacity;
- focus on community-led initiatives that use relevant local content;
- involve women in planning and use;
- encourage long-term planning and policies;
- seek cooperative partnerships;
- combine old and new technologies.

A key to strengthening health and other social systems is to improve the skills of the people within those systems. Increased effort is going into improving information technology skills. But there is also a need to improve information management, repackaging, and communication skills, as well as building basic organizational capacity. This means making a significant time and resource commitment to invest in training and in "understanding people's problems before applying technology to solve them" (Chetley, 2001; Peizer, 2000).

A U.S. Peace Corps project in Gambia found the process of ensuring sustainability was "more difficult and time consuming than bringing in the actual hardware." The lesson learned was that development "is done by building the human resource base, and ensuring that the community feels included every step of the way" (Chetley, 2001; Soh, 2001).

More attention needs to be paid to innovative ways of applying ICTs to the specific information needs of communities and local groups. That includes focusing on building local skills to encourage the process of local appropriation and reinforcing traditional information communication networks (Chetley, 2001).

It is important to keep an open mind about the kinds of ICTs that are likely to be most appropriate for these purposes. There is a tendency at present to center discussion of information and communications technologies around the Internet and to channel development assistance largely toward facilitating access to it. But cutting-edge applications are not always what people need most. In some cases, Internet use may prove too expensive or too difficult for local people to maintain, and thus be unsustainable. And in others, the Internet is simply not the best medium for supporting local socioeconomic and political progress (Alcantara, 2001).

When designing ICT programs in developing countries, several constraints must be explicitly taken into account. Thus, at the international level, discussion of possibilities to use the Internet for improving trade and employment opportunities in low-income countries must be accompanied by a frank evaluation of impediments associated with the current global financial and trade situation. If the surrounding context for proposed innovation is not sufficiently analyzed, and if remedies for pressing economic problems are not addressed, many well-meaning efforts will have short lives and minimal results (Alcantara, 2001).

ICT IN THE CONTEXT OF THE PEPFAR INITIATIVE

Recent studies have shown the feasibility of treating HIV/AIDS in developing countries. ICT systems can be effectively used to track clinical outcomes, laboratory tests, and drug supplies, and create reports for funding agencies. Development and evaluation of practical, low cost clinical information systems should be strongly considered when rolling out HIV treatment in developing countries. However, utilizing ICTs in some developing countries is challenging, especially due to the lack of telecommunication infrastructure, which is considered a barrier to successful HIV treatment programs in resource-constrained settings. Different approaches can be implemented for managing clinical and laboratory information in developing countries.

In the context of the PEPFAR initiative, ICT can support workforce expansion, including patient screening and rapid assessment, diagnostic tools, ARV management, community outreach, patient tracking, demographic surveys, distance learning, etc. This is, in fact, a wide spectrum of applications, and some priorities have to be set in order to make it feasible and cost-effective, keeping in mind that both local professionals as well as professionals sent from abroad to work on this initiative should benefit from ICT tools that will be put in place.

Access to the Internet and bandwidth in several developing countries, especially in Africa, are limited and expensive, compared to the rates charged in developed countries. This is mainly attributable to the lack of local resources and reliable telecommunication networks. Connection to the Internet is established through some available technologies that use either wired links, such as dial-up and leased lines (which are not reliable in most of the African countries) or wireless links, such as satellite, radio links, or Wi-Fi. Wireless links and mobile phones have been widely used in African countries, as they do not need to rely on the local wired telephone network.

Additional difficulties often relate to unreliable electrical infrastructure that may render a site without electrical power for five or more hours every day. Some rural areas in Uganda, for instance, have power outages twice a day. Generators or power supplies have to be implemented at the sites to assure that power will be available for the IT equipment as well as for the freezers that store blood samples, when applicable.

Security measures have also to be taken due to the sensitive nature of the data and to ensure confidentiality of people living with HIV/AIDS. A comprehensive data backup and disaster recovery plan have to be in place to restore system information in case of loss of the primary data.

One of the major challenges of the PEPFAR initiative is that it includes several countries with different realities regarding culture, available resources, and technology infrastructure. It is clear that there is not a unique solution that can be applied for all PEPFAR countries, as several barriers and difficulties have to be overcome in order to implement a site-specific IT infrastructure. The approaches, solutions, and tools have to be adapted to each reality in order to make a wise use of the PEPFAR funds as well as each country's resources.

Many countries in sub-Saharan Africa, for instance, present a unique set of difficulties and barriers to effective ICT implementation. Perhaps the foremost obstacle is the lack of a sufficient and reliable telecommunication infrastructure. This often forces applications that require consistent connectivity to incur high fees to bypass in-country networks and local telecom connections that fail frequently because of inadequate maintenance and mismanagement.

Other problems arise from government monopolies and excessive regulation, as in Kenya, where radio frequency and satellite licensing formalities can delay solution implementations by months or years. Kenya and other African countries currently route out-of-country Internet traffic through a central government monopoly, which slows down transmissions considerably. Government bureaucracy in general is often slow, and new technologies are constantly prevented from adoption because local authorities fail to "approve" new technologies in a timely manner. The UN organizations, the U.S. Embassy, some NGOs, and most private banks have special license to uplink in Kenya, by-passing the government Internet provider.

In places where Internet access and bandwidth are not widely available, or not cheap, standalone systems can be implemented to avoid real-time data transmission. However, some aspects have to be taken into account:

• Is there any interest to have data from all PEPFAR countries in a central database in the United States, for instance? If so, is there a need for readily access to the data generated at the remote sites? How often should the data be updated?

• How many different sites (health centers, hospitals and clinics) will be running ICT systems? Do they need to be integrated or will they run standalone systems and databases?

Answers to these questions lead to different ICT approaches as well as different implementation costs. It is true that in some locations, it is possible to establish strategic partnerships with local organizations, hospitals, or universities in order to share IT infrastructure, reducing costs while at the same time preserving data privacy.

Nowadays, standalone systems without communication with central databases or integration with counterpart systems do not accomplish much. When data has to be transferred to central databases, different offline solutions can be used, depending on technologies and bandwidth available, as well as cost and service reliability. In this case, data can be stored in local databases and data updates are transferred to central databases during off-hours, for instance. This is a wise and cost effective way to implement ICT systems in resource-constrained settings.

Other approaches use online systems across the Internet (web-based systems or client-server applications) or through virtual private networks. The advantages of online systems are: they allow for swift data acquisition and reliable data transfer to the central databases; they allow scientists to access clinical data faster; they prevent blood samples and Case Report Forms from having to be physically transported from rural areas to the main cities for data entry; they allow a laboratory to process lab exams more rapidly and confirm sample identity; they give local professionals an opportunity to exchange information quickly and to be up-to-date on research studies and news related to the field study; and they also increase the local capacity of the sites. Staff at clinical sites also benefit from access to the latest research information on the Internet, e-mail communication, and real-time clinical research data. It also helps to reduce the isolation of researchers and professionals working in the field by enabling them to be in constant contact with other professionals and exchange information and results faster.

Judicious ICT implementation allows for swift data processing and assures that valuable and accurate information will be available to health professionals, so that they can make critical decisions in a timely fashion, especially those related to serious adverse events (Lima et al., 2004), when applicable.

Investing in developing country's ICT infrastructure has important externalities that benefit local communities and economies by increasing the demand for ICT-related services, facilitating the training of individuals in computers and networking, as well as increasing their ICT capacity for use in other development initiatives.

Vital to finding solutions for disparate sites are detailed assessments that take into account both the needs of the prospective site and the local and national climate for ICT. For instance, it would be ill-advised to install a system that could not be supported by local talent. This is often successfully countered by providing additional training and support to otherwise capable IT consultants and, when necessary, assistance may be provided from abroad, particularly from U.S. participants of the PEPFAR initiative.

Finally, conducting clinical trials in resource-constrained settings almost always presents challenges of getting appropriate technology to remote sites quickly, accelerating slow medical panels in granting regulatory approval, when applicable, and assuring that proper steps are taken to protect patient privacy and site security. These technologies, while sometimes challenging and difficult to implement, are central to coordinate the efforts of the PEPFAR initiative.

The following sections provide some examples of information systems to support HIV treatment in developing countries (Fraser et al., 2004).

Stand Alone Databases

• The Brazilian public health system currently delivers antiretroviral treatment to more than 148,000 patients—by far the largest group in the developing world. The "Computerized System for the Control of Drug Logistics (SICLOM)" (Veloso et al., 2000) is an Internet based drug management program developed to support treatment and is considered a "key factor helping to overcome logistical challenges to delivery of antiretroviral treatment in Brazil." It connects to a central server to update its records.

• The Mosoriot medical record in Kenya has been heavily used for general medical care in one hospital for more than 2 years and was recently extended to support HIV treatment at Moi University. It was developed using Microsoft Access; data are entered from a paper record. A web-based version is under development.

• The Children's Hospital in Lilongwe, Malawi, has made heavy use of a touch-screen medical record system for more than 2 years. Developed by Gerry Douglas, this system runs on a local network and is built using Microsoft SQL server and Visual Basic. Doctors, nurses, and other staff enter all data, including drug orders. It is being extended to collect data on HIV patients.

• The Cuban health ministry has a Microsoft Access database system called SIDATRAT that registers general patient data, clinical data, opportunistic infections, staging, viral load and CD4 cell count, treatment, side effects, drug resistance, and drug adherence. It includes the more than 5,000 people diagnosed with HIV in Cuba since 1986.

• A team at the U.S. Department of Health and Human Services led by John Milberg has developed the Careware system (using Microsoft Access). It provides comprehensive tools for tracking HIV patients and their treatment. Currently used in more than 300 U.S. health centers and hospitals, it was deployed in Uganda in October 2003. An internet accessible version is under development. Software is available free at http://hab.hrsa.gov/careware.

• FUCHIA was developed by Epicentre, the epidemiology group of Médecins Sans Frontières, to support their HIV treatment projects. It supports clinical care and long term follow up of patients, including scheduling of visits, and includes data on drugs and certain investigations and generates some reports. It was developed using Microsoft Access and the Delphi programming language, and the software is available free at www.epicentre.msf.org.

Internet-Based Medical Record Systems

• The PIH-EMR system was created to support the management of drug resistant tuberculosis in Peru. This system was built using the Linux operating system, Apache web server, Tomcat Java Servlet engine, and Oracle database. It supports clinical care, logistics such as assessment of drug requirements, and research studies. Heavily used for more than 2 years, most data are entered from paper forms, with nurse entry of drug orders now implemented in some sites.

• The HIV-EMR is an information system and medical record to support HIV treatment in rural Haiti. The central database is hosted on a server in Boston, Massachusetts. Clinical data forms include demographic data, clinical assessment, laboratory investigations, and social circumstances. The system includes a library of web page analyses, developed for a related project, that simplify searches for patient groups based on characteristics such as age, drug regimen, and laboratory results. Other pages generate graphs and tables and allow data to be downloaded to statistical analysis packages. More information can be found at http://bmj.com/cgi/content/full/329/7475/1142.

• Voxiva developed an application named Alerta that enables health officials to conduct real-time disease surveillance and rapidly respond to disease outbreaks, even in the most remote regions of the world where access to modern communications devices is limited. Alerta is a solution that combines the Internet and the telephone to extend the benefits of software applications to people without access to the Internet. The solution includes a web site for authorized users, telephone access and data entry, and a database that stores data submitted by both phone and web. The system is operational 24 hours a day, 7 days a week. More information can be found at www.voxiva.net.

• The Brazilian STD/AIDS Programme has developed the "System of Control of Laboratory Exams (SISCEL)" (Lima et al., 2000) to take into account the needs of the Brazilian Network of Public Health Laboratories, which carries out CD4+/CD8+ count and viral load exams in 94 health centers throughout the country. SISCEL links all laboratories via Internet and is meant to manage, process, follow up, and analyze its CD4 and viral load test results, as well as to optimize the exam-requesting and result-issuing procedures. The system has been designed to run online with quality, including security mechanisms.

Web-Based Collaboration and Telemedicine Systems (Not Specifically for HIV)

• The RAFT project permits remote collaboration, case discussion, and data sharing over low bandwidth networks between Geneva University Hospitals and Bamako, Mali. The collaboration is being extended to other French West-African countries. It is built using Linux and other open source software.

• The IPATH server allows image sharing in pathology and radiology and is being used in South Africa and the Pacific as well as Switzerland. It is built with open source software and is available free at www.sourceforge.net.

• Telemedmail is a secure email and web based telemedicine system under evaluation in South Africa and Peru; it was built using Java and open source software and is available free at www.sourceforge.net.

• Satellife is using the cell phone network in Uganda to transfer data to a central site. Local healthcare workers collect data on Palm Pilots and then connect to a local, battery powered server called a Wide Ray Jack. This server allows data to be sent to and from a central database via a cell phone modem. More information is at http://pda.healthnet.org.

• The International AIDS Vaccine Initiative (IAVI) performs multi-center HIV vaccine clinical trials in resource-constrained settings, mainly in Africa, utilizing centralized databases for data management. IAVI implements efficient and cost-effective telecommunication infrastructure at the sites, to allow data transfer through the Internet to central databases, using radio links, leased lines, or satellite connections. Online (web-based systems) and offline solutions (Datafax) are used, depending on technologies and bandwidth available, as well as cost and service reliability. Security measures are taken due to the sensitive nature of the data and to ensure confidentiality of trial participants. More information about IAVI's work can be seen at www.iavi.org.

FINAL CONSIDERATIONS AND QUESTIONS

Realistic Goals and Appropriate Assessment

ICTs cannot stand alone in most, if not all, health programs and initiatives. Conducting an appropriate assessment to assess the potential benefit that ICTs may bring to the project or initiative remains central to an effective and sustainable implementation.

ICT assessment should occur in the formative research or communication analysis phase of planning programs.

Key Assessment Questions:

1. In what ways can ICT benefit the prospective project?
2. Will ICT serve a communicative (e.g., websites, training) and/or backend function (e.g., data collection, resource monitoring)?
3. What are the most critical applications that should be implemented?
4. What are the prospective limitations, liabilities, and risks of using ICT in a particular application? How might they be mitigated?
5. How many and what cities of the PEPFAR countries will be included in the initiative, and what type of information system and database are needed?
6. How many people will be included in the database, and what is their geographic distribution?
7. What type of information system should be managed? Clinical and/or laboratorial?
8. What are the training needs?

Key Assessment Points:

1. Evaluation of telecommunication infrastructure
2. Availability, cost, and reliability of bandwidth
3. Evaluation of local capacity and establishment of partnerships
4. Analysis of social and political situation
5. Privacy and confidentiality
6. Security mechanisms
7. Condition of electrical power supply (implementation of generator, UPS, etc.)
8. Data backup and disaster recovery

Sustainability and Implementation Success

Oftentimes the latest ICTs are not the best solutions to implement, it is not uncommon for program developers to overlook older more tested and more supported ICTs in the name of being "high tech."

Prospective ICTs should be measured against original project goals. Does the ICT fulfill the given need?

The sustainability of a particular ICT has technical, social, and administrative dimensions.

Key Sustainability Questions:

1. Can the ICT applications be supported adequately by local personnel?

2. Are there sufficient stakeholders (of the ICT) within the project? Have the stakeholders contributed and/or assisted in the implementation of the ICT?

3. Will the implemented ICT infrastructure and systems increase the capacity of the sites and bring contributions to the local professionals?

REFERENCES

Alcantara CH. 2001. *The Development Divide in a Digital Age.* Geneva, Switzerland: United Nations Research Institute for Social Development (UNRISD).

Chetley A. 2001. Improving health, fighting poverty: the role of information and communication technology (ICT). *Exchange* (1). [Online]. Available: http://www.healthcomms.org/pdf/findings1.pdf [accessed March 22, 2005].

Delgadillo K, Borja R. 1999. *Learning Lessons from telecentres in Latin America and the Caribbean.* Ottowa, Canada: International Development Research Centre (IDRC).

Fraser HS, Jazayeri D, Nevil P, Karacaoglu Y, Farmer PE, Lyon E, Fawzi MK, Leandre F, Choi SS, Mukherjee JS. 2004. An information system and medical record to support HIV treatment in rural Haiti. *BMJ* 329(7475):1142–1146.

Lima R, Dantas MCS, Vilela WT, et al. 2000 (July). *SISCEL: A Nationwide System for Managing CD4 and Viral Load Exams in the Brazilian Network of Public Health Laboratories.* Presented at the XIII International AIDS Conference, Durban, South Africa.

Lima R, Branch G, Muluubya A, et al. 2004 (July). *Implementing an Information Technology (IT) Infrastructure for HIV Vaccine Clinical Trials in Resource-Constrained Settings.* Presented at the XV International AIDS Conference, Bangkok, Thailand.

Peizer J. 2000 (June). *Bridging the Digital Divide: First You Need the Bridge.* [Online]. Available: http://www.mediachannel.org/views/oped/peizer.shtml [accessed March 22, 2005].

Soh C. 2001 (April). *Resurrecting the Dinosaur: Creating Networks to Recycle ICT Hardware.* [Online]. Available: http://www.iconnect-online.org/Stories/Story.import69 [accessed March 22, 2005].

Storey M. 1999. *Information and Communication Technology.* [Online]. Available: http://www.aiha.com/index.jsp?sid=1&id=1279&pid=4739 [accessed March 22, 2005].

Veloso V, Sudo E, Lima R, et al. 2000 (July). *Promoting the Rational Use of Antiretrovirals Through a Computer Aided System for the Logistical Control of Aids Medications in Brazil.* Presented at the XIII International AIDS Conference, Durban, South Africa.

Appendix G

Attributes of Governmental and Nongovernmental Organizational Models for the Potential Administration of the Global Health Service

SAMPLING OF ORGANIZATIONAL MODEL ATTRIBUTES

TABLE G-1 Governmental Organizational Models

Government Agency	Attributes
CDC Epidemic Intelligence Service (EIS) http://www.cdc.gov/eis	• Headquartered at CDC, an agency of the Department of Health and Human Services (DHHS) and receives its budget and congressional oversight through DHHS. • Employs qualified personnel for 2-year positions. • International work can be part of a 2-year service, but service is never completely overseas. • EIS officers are placed within CDC or a similar agency. • Have 20 field programs to support international efforts. • 130 current EIS officers that are placed according to the needs of a specific location. • Epidemiologic investigations can be related to HIV/AIDS.
CDC Global AIDS Program (GAP) http://www.cdc.gov/nchstp/od/gap/default.htm	• CDC is an agency of the DHHS and receives its budget and congressional oversight through DHHS. • GAP works under the direction of the Office of the Global AIDS coordinator. • Deploy and employ experienced staff for 2-year terms. • Maintain offices abroad including support staff. • Active in 25 countries including all PEPFAR countries. • Programs include addressing opportunistic infections, TB, and other STIs. Focus on prevention and surveillance.
Health Resources and Services Administration (HRSA) http://www.hrsa.gov	• HRSA is an agency of the DHHS and receives its budget and congressional oversight through DHHS. • Programs were domestic until recently (intradepartmental delegation of authority from CDC) but it is unclear if they have the capacity to support volunteers overseas. • One of their strategies is to provide support to developing countries to rapidly expand the pool of trained providers, managers, and allied health staff to improve HIV/AIDS, TB, and malaria services. In addition they

TABLE G-1 Continued

Government Agency	Attributes
	conduct training activities to support human capacity; strengthen the capacity to collect data and monitor and evaluate data on health care services; and establish partnerships that support human resource capacity development.
Indian Health Service (IHS) http://www.ihs.gov	• IHS is an agency of the DHHS and receives its budget and congressional oversight through DHHS. • Provides health services to approximately 1.5 million American Indians and Alaska Natives who belong to more than 557 federally recognized tribes in 35 states. • Recruit every discipline involved in providing health care, social, and environmental health services. • Offer recruitment incentives such as loan repayment and scholarships to attract professionals. • HIV/AIDS services may be included.
National Health Service Corps (NHSC) http://nhsc.bhpr.hrsa.gov	• NHSC is part of the Health Resources and Services Administration which is an agency of the DHHS and receives its budget and congressional oversight through DHHS. • Deploy highly skilled health professionals (placement limited to clinicians) to underserved areas in the United States for 2-3 years service. • No international mandate or experience. • Offer recruitment incentives such as loan repayment to attract professionals. • Primary care provided by deployed clinicians could include HIV/AIDS care and treatment.
Peace Corps www.peacecorps.gov	• The Peace Corps is an independent agency within the executive branch of the U.S. Government. The Peace Corps' annual budget is determined each year by the congressional budget and appropriations process, and is part of the foreign operations budget. • The Senate Foreign Relations Committee is charged with general oversight of the activities and programs of the Peace Corps, and the House Committee on International Relations serves a similar function.

continued

TABLE G-1 Continued

Government Agency	Attributes
	• Recruit and deploy volunteers (nonsalaried) for 2-year service.
	• Deploy skilled volunteers for specific assignments (usually 6 months) under Crisis Corps.
	• Maintain at least one main office in every active country including support staff.
	• Currently active in 72 countries, including all PEPFAR focus countries.
	• 20 percent of the current 7,733 volunteers work on health and HIV/AIDS.
United States Agency for International Development (USAID) http://www.usaid.gov	• USAID is an independent federal government agency that receives overall foreign policy guidance from the secretary of state.
	• Employs skilled staff overseas.
	• Works in all of the PEPFAR countries.
	• Maintains offices in over 80 countries around the world including support staff.
	• Works on HIV/AIDS issues under PEPFAR.
Volunteers for Prosperity http://volunteersforprosperity.gov	• Is part of USA Freedom Corps.
	• Supports international voluntary service but does not deploy.
	• No capacity to support volunteers or overseas workers.
	• Provides recognition to volunteers.
	• Has about 200 for profit and nonprofit organizations on website.
	• Supports U.S. development initiatives including PEPFAR.

TABLE G-2 Nongovernmental Organizational Models

Nongovernment Agency	Attributes
American International Health Alliance (AIHA) http://www.aiha.com	• Focus on twinning and are recipients of Twinning Center award from HRSA. • Participants in twinning projects include a variety of health professionals depending on the need of the international partner and the specific project. • No experience with long term deployment of volunteers but plan to deploy volunteers linked to PEPFAR twinning projects for 3–6 months. • Volunteers receive no compensation but do receive reimbursement for travel expenses. • No experience in PEPFAR countries. • Experience addressing HIV/AIDS through twinning partnerships.
Catholic Medical Mission Board (CMMB) http://www.cmmb.org	• Focus on addressing immediate needs by providing care and building capacity through training. • Places only experienced, licensed professionals. • Volunteer service usually one year or more with limited available placements ranging from 1–6 months. • Has a program that provides physicians traveling abroad with medical supplies. • Experience in some, but not all PEPFAR countries. • Addresses HIV/AIDS.
Health Volunteers Overseas (HVO) http://www.hvousa.org	• Focus on training, not providing care. • Service is usually 1 month but shorter assignments of 2 weeks are sometimes feasible as are longer assignments of 3–6 months. • Supports over 60 projects in more than 25 countries. • Deploys specific specialties of highly skilled professionals. • Volunteers pay their own way, but HVO lists some funding opportunities on their website. • Addresses HIV/AIDS.

continued

TABLE G-2 Continued

Nongovernment Agency	Attributes
International Center for Equal Healthcare Access (ICEHA) http://www.iceha.org	• Focus on infectious diseases with an emphasis on HIV/AIDS. • Deploy physicians and nurses to improve clinical skills of local health care providers by using a method of clinical mentoring and informal didactic training. • Deploy physician assistants, and pharmacists to work as a team with volunteer physicians. • Volunteer service is a minimum of 2 months, not usually long term. • Of the PEPFAR countries, have experience in Côte d'Ivoire, Nigeria, and Vietnam. • Volunteers do not provide care but only build local clinical expertise. • Volunteers donate their time. • Addresses HIV/AIDS.
JHPIEGO http://www.jhpiego.org	• Focus on building capacity, promoting sound health policies, learning innovatively, developing networks, and promoting best practices. • Hire local staff, third country nationals, expatriots, or consultants. • Works in 37 countries, has offices in 14 countries including many of the PEPFAR focus countries. • Addresses HIV/AIDS and close ties to Johns Hopkins University provide easy access to expertise from internationally known leaders in the field.
UMCOR http://gbgm-umc.org/umcor	• Work in 88 countries, 20 of which have large projects. • Deploys about 187,000 volunteers a year (both domestically and internationally) in teams of 10. • Volunteers pay their own way. • Deployments range from months to years. • Qualifications vary with assignment. • Some assignments may address HIV/AIDS.

Appendix H

Biographies

COMMITTEE MEMBERS

Fitzhugh Mullan, M.D. (Chair), is a contributing editor of the journal *Health Affairs* and a clinical professor of pediatrics and public health at the George Washington University. He is a member of the medical staff at the Upper Cardozo Community Health Center in Washington, D.C. Dr. Mullan graduated from Harvard University and from the University of Chicago Medical School. In 1972 he was commissioned in the U.S. Public Health Service and went to work as one of the first physicians in the National Health Service Corps. From 1977 through 1981 he served as director of the program followed by tours as a senior medical officer at the National Institutes of Health and, in 1984–1985, as the Secretary of Health and Environment for the state of New Mexico. He was appointed director of the Bureau of Health Professions in 1990 and to the rank of Assistant Surgeon General (Rear Admiral) in 1991. In subsequent years, he served on both the President's Task Force on Health Care Reform and the Council on Graduate Medical Education. Dr. Mullan retired from the Public Health Service in 1996. Dr. Mullan has written widely for professional and general audiences, including his books *Plagues and Politics: The Story of the United States Public Health Service*, and *Big Doctoring in America: Profiles in Primary Care*. Dr. Mullan is the Founding President of the National Coalition for Cancer Survivorship. He serves as Vice-Chair of the Board of Trustees of the National Health Museum.

Michele Barry, M.D., F.A.C.P., is a Professor of Medicine and Global Public Health at Yale University where she is the Director of Yale's Office

231

of International Health. She also serves as the health consultant for the Ford Foundation overseas programs. As codirector for more than 20 years of Yale/Johnson and Johnson Physician Scholar Award program she has sent more than 800 physicians overseas to underserved areas. As a past president of the American Society of Tropical Medicine and Hygiene, she led an educational initiative in tropical medicine and travelers health which culminated in diploma courses in tropical medicine both in the United States and overseas, as well as a U.S. certification exam. She has written extensively in the areas of clinical tropical diseases, refugee health, and ethical dilemmas of overseas research. Dr. Barry has lived overseas on projects in Ecuador, Zimbabwe, Tanzania, Haiti, and South Africa.

Jane Carter, M.B.B.S., F.R.C.P.(C.), is Head of the Clinical Services Program for the African Medical and Research Foundation, located in Nairobi, Kenya. As Head of the Laboratory Program, Dr. Carter pilots her own single-engine Cessna and flies to 80 remote villages in East Africa to help establish outreach services or set up a lab. Dr. Carter, one of the foundation's "Flying Doctors," has a medical practice that covers more than 1.5 million square kilometers. In addition to her establishing outreach services, Dr. Carter is responsible for developing and supervising clinical and laboratory diagnostic services. She also coordinates with African ministries of health and other health care agencies to develop training methods and learning materials, and does operational research into diagnostic systems development and diagnostic methodologies. Born in Calcutta, Dr. Carter spent her early childhood in developing countries such as Pakistan and Sri Lanka and later attended boarding school in England. She later earned a medical degree at the Royal Free Hospital in London. Dr. Carter did her residency training in general internal medicine at the University of Toronto, where she later specialized in clinical hematology.

Lincoln Chen, M.D., M.P.H., is the Director of the Global Equity Center at Harvard Kennedy School of Government. Previously he has served as the Executive Vice President for Strategy at the Rockefeller Foundation, and as a member of the Board of Trustees Committee on Future Strategies chairs or directs programs in global philanthropy, such as the Program Venture Experiment and the Bellagio Committee. Prior to joining the Rockefeller Foundation, Dr. Chen was the Director of the University-wide Harvard Center for Population and Development Studies and the Taro Takemi Professor of International Health at the Harvard School of Public Health. From 1981–1987, Dr. Chen was the Representative of the Ford Foundation in India, and in 1973–1980, he worked for the Ford Foundation both on its staff and seconded as Scientific Director of the International Center for Diarrheal Disease Research in Bangladesh. Dr. Chen has more than 100 publications on world social development, especially in health, population, and food and nutrition.

Gary Gunderson, M.Div, D.Min, is Director of the Interfaith Health Program (IHP) of the Rollins School of Public Health, Emory University. Dr. Gunderson is the author of *Deeply Woven Roots* (Fortress, 1997), exploring the strengths of religious congregations as agents in building healthy communities, and *Playing to Our Strengths* (Carter Center, 1997), examining the opportunities and challenges in the realignment of religious health assets such as hospitals and the new foundations. He has also published many articles and speeches. He is the program chair for the American Public Health Association caucus on Faith Community and Public Health, consultant to the United Methodist Bishop's Initiative on Children and Poverty, member of the Board of Directors of Heifer Project International and the Atlanta Committee for UNICEF, and co-chair of Oakhurst Baptist Building Fund. Gunderson is an ordained American Baptist minister educated at Wake Forest University (history), Emory University (M.Div.) and Interdenominational Theological Center (D.Min.). Gunderson was the founder and editor of *Seeds* magazine, which won international recognition for excellence in coverage of hunger and international development. He led a private company, USAfrica, for 5 years, establishing joint venture projects and consulting with governments in Africa. He has served as Honorary Consul for the country of Burkina Faso, West Africa, since 1988.

Barry Kistnasamy, M.B.Ch.B., M.Med., is a specialist in Community Health with further training in Health Economics and Planning (York, UK) and Environmental and Occupational Health (University of Michigan, Ann Arbor). He is currently the program manager for HIV/AIDS in the Department of Community Health at the Nelson R. Mandela School of Medicine in Durban, South Africa. Before becoming the program manager for HIV/AIDS, he served as Dean of Medicine of the Nelson R. Mandela School of Medicine, as Deputy Director General of Health, Welfare and Environment in the Northern Cape, and as advisor to the Minister of Health in KwaZulu-Natal. He received an M.B.Ch.B. and an M.Med. (Community Health) from the University of Natal. He has also studied Health Economics and Planning in York (UK), Occupational and Environmental Health in Michigan, and Health Leadership in Cambridge (UK). Dr. Kistnasamy contributed to health policy development in South Africa (Occupational Health, Health Financing and Human Resources) and has been involved with Health System transformation over the last 20 years. He also serves in various nongovernmental organizations and professional and academic bodies in South Africa.

Ronaldo Lima, M.Sc., is Senior Director of Information Technology for the International AIDS Vaccine Initiative. A native of Brazil, Mr. Lima has a Bachelor of Science in electronic engineering and a master's degree in computer networks from Federal University of Rio de Janeiro, Brazil. Besides engineering, he has also been involved in AIDS advocacy since 1991 as president of an AIDS community-based organization named Grupo Pela Vidda, in Rio de Janeiro. In 1999, Mr. Lima was invited to work for the Brazilian National AIDS Program in Brasilia as the head of the Information Technology Department where he employed his different experiences in information technology as well as in the AIDS field. In this position he led 23 technical consultants in advancing the implementation of three nationwide information systems. He has also been involved particularly with AIDS vaccine advocacy during the last 3 years, being one of the community representatives in the Brazilian National AIDS Vaccine Committee. In 2000, Mr. Lima moved to the United States to work as an information technology consultant for an American company located in California. In September 2001, Mr. Lima moved to New York to join IAVI and, once more, is bringing together his backgrounds in information technology, management, and vaccine advocacy.

Leslie Mancuso, Ph.D., R.N., is CEO of JHPIEGO, where she provides strategic direction and coordination of JHPIEGO's major programs and awards, directs the corporate management of program, technical, and administrative operations, and manages and guides JHPIEGO's business development activities. Prior to serving as CEO, Dr. Mancuso was Acting Chief Executive Officer and Chief Operating Officer, and later served as a Vice President for Project HOPE, a $100 million not-for-profit organization active in the training of health care professionals and the provision of medicines and medical supplies in more than 30 low-income countries worldwide. The international health community recognizes Dr. Mancuso as a leader in the field because of her pioneering work in neonatal and pediatric care. Under her leadership, Dr. Mancuso provides her staff of 400 with a vision for how JHPIEGO can maximize both public and private sector resources to create sustainable health networks throughout the world. JHPIEGO works with many international organizations, including HealthNet International, UNICEF, the World Health Organization (WHO), the U.S. Centers for Disease Control and Prevention (CDC), and the United States Agency for International Development (USAID).

MG (Retired) William L. Moore, Jr., M.D., served as Chief Medical Executive, Department of Veterans Affairs, and Clinical Professor of Medicine, Division of Infectious Diseases, Vanderbilt University Medical Center. Dr. Moore is a nationally known infectious diseases physician-epidemiologist who has authored/co-authored more than 40 scientific articles in peer-reviewed journals. Dr. Moore retired from the U.S. Army at the rank of Major General. His assignments included Vice Commander, Headquarters, Joint Military Medical Command; Commander, Brooke Army Medical Center; and Commander, U.S. Army Medical Department Center and School. As Commander of the U.S. Army Medical Department Center and School, Dr. Moore oversaw DoD-wide programs for training combat medics and other professional extenders for work in low resource settings. Early in his career he trained Special Forces medics and also directed Army AIDS programs. Prior to his position with the Department of Veterans Affairs, he was State Epidemiologist and Director of Communicable and Environmental Disease Services Section of the Tennessee Department of Health. His primary areas of expertise include infectious diseases, sexually transmitted diseases, epidemiology, military medicine, and public health. Dr. Moore is board certified in internal medicine and infectious diseases, and a fellow of the American College of Physicians and the Infectious Diseases Society of America. Dr. Moore has served as a member on many local, state, and national panels and committees. Dr. Moore's extensive background in military medicine and his diverse expertise in infectious diseases, hospital administration, epidemiology, and public health contribute greatly to the Board's ability to provide recommendations to DoD on a variety of important health issues.

Andre-Jacques Neusy, M.D., DTM&H, is the founder and director of the Center for Global Health at NYU School of Medicine, dedicated to shaping new interdisciplinary education and capacity development strategies for health and health-allied professionals. Dr. Neusy was raised in Congo-Zaire where he completed his premedical education. He obtained his medical degree and a certificate in Tropical Medicine and Hygiene at the Free University of Brussels School of Medicine. He joined the faculty of New York University's School of Medicine in 1975. Dr. Neusy returned numerous times to Africa to serve as health coordinator in development and disaster settings. In 1994, he led the health team of the International Rescue Committee (IRC), responding to the humanitarian crisis in the aftermath of the genocide in Rwanda. A technical advisor to its Health Unit, Dr. Neusy has worked for IRC, a $148 million not-for-profit organization involved in emergency relief and rehabilitation in 25 countries, in Eastern Zaire, Macedonia, and Kosovo. Committed to strengthening global human resources for health, Dr. Neusy serves as advisor to the Ministry of Health and the National University of Rwanda. President of the International Health Medical Education Consortium, he has lectured on disaster management and global health-related issues at various institutions.

Lieutenant General James B. Peake, MC, USA, is a graduate of the military academy at West Point and has held a wide variety of important positions in the U.S. Army, culminating in his appointment September 22, 2000, as Army Surgeon General and Commander of the U.S. Army Medical Command, Fort Sam Houston, Texas. Previous key assignments include: Commander, U.S. Army Medical Department Center and School, and Installation Commander, Fort Sam Houston, Texas; Deputy Commander, U.S. Army Medical Command, Fort Sam Houston, Texas; Commanding General, Madigan Army Medical Center/Northwest Health Service Support Activity, Tacoma, Washington; Commanding General, 44th Medical Brigade/Corps Surgeon, XVIII Airborne Corps, Fort Bragg, North Carolina; Deputy Director, Professional Services/Chief, Consultant, Office of the Surgeon General, Falls Church, Virgnia; Commander, 18th Medical Command and 121st Evacuation Hospital/Command Surgeon, Seoul, Korea; Deputy Commander for Clinical Services, Tripler Army Medical Center, Honolulu, Hawaii; Assistant Chief, Cardiothoracic Surgery, Brooke Army Medical Center, Fort Sam Houston, Texas; Staff General Surgeon/Chief, General Surgery Clinic, DeWitt Army Hospital, Fort Belvoir, Virginia; and General Surgery Resident, Brooke Army Medical Center, Fort Sam Houston, Texas.

Christina Polyak, M.P.H., is currently a medical student at the University of Maryland. Ms. Polyak previously operated as an epidemiologist with the Centers for Disease Control and Prevention and the Department of Defense's Global Emerging Infections System at the Walter Reed Army Institute of Research. Her work has included extended field assignments in Kenya and Malawi. She has published and presented extensively in the field of epidemiology and is a member of the American Society of Tropical Medicine and Hygiene, the International Society of Travel Medicine, and the American Medical Student Association. Ms. Polyak received her Bachelor of Science and Master's in Public Health at Johns Hopkins University.

Marla Salmon, ScD., R.N., currently serves as Professor and Dean, Nell Hodgson Woodruff School of Nursing and Professor at the Rollins School of Public Health of Emory University. Prior to joining Emory, Dr. Salmon served as professor and graduate dean of the School of Nursing at the University of Pennsylvania, where she was responsible for both master's and doctoral nursing programs. Prior to her role at the University of Pennsylvania, Dr. Salmon served as director of the Division of Nursing for the United States Department of Health and Human Services; Professor and Chair of Public Health Nursing in the School of Public Health at the University of North Carolina; and Head of the Public Health Nursing Program at the University of Minnesota. Her areas of teaching and research include health policy and administration, public health nursing, and health workforce development. Dr. Salmon is the author of numerous publications in these areas. Dr. Salmon has worked with a number of international organizations, including the World Health Organization, the Pan American Health Organization and the W. K. Kellogg Foundation. In addition, Dr. Salmon has consulted with governments and organizations outside of the United States and served as a member of the U.S. Delegation to the World Health Assembly. Dr. Salmon is the former Chair of the World Health Organization's Global Advisory Group on Nursing and Midwifery. Dr. Salmon received her doctoral degree from Johns Hopkins University School of Hygiene and Public Health, holds degrees in nursing and political science from the University of Portland and is the recipient of two honorary degrees. Dr. Salmon has also been a Fellow in the W. K. Kellogg National Fellowship Program and the Hubert H. Humphrey Institute of Public Affairs.

Robert Schooley, M.D., is Professor and Head of the Division of Infectious Diseases at the University of California, San Diego. He has served as Chair of the NIH's AIDS and Related Retrovirus 1 Study Section and as Chair of the Executive Committee of the NIAID's AIDS Clinical Trials Group (ACTG). He currently serves as International Program Liaison for the ACTG. Dr. Schooley is a Member of the AIDS Treatment Guidelines Panels of the Department of Health and Human Services and of the International AIDS Society–USA. He is also a member of the American Association for the Advancement of Science; American Society for Clinical Investigation; American Society for Microbiology; Clinical Immunology Society; and Association of American Physicians and is a Fellow of the Infectious Disease Society. His research interests are in the areas of viral pathogenesis and therapy.

Harrison Spencer, M.D., M.P.H., is President and CEO of the Association of Schools of Public Health. Before that, he was Dean of the London School of Hygiene and Tropical Medicine. He has also served as Dean of Tulane School of Public Health and Chief of the parasitic disease branch at the CDC. Dr. Spencer received his bachelor's degree from Haverford College and his medical degree from Johns Hopkins University School of Medicine. He holds a M.P.H. in epidemiology from Berkeley, as well as a diploma in tropical medicine and hygiene from the London School of Hygiene and Tropical Medicine (DTM&H). He is a member of many expert committees of the World Health Organization and many professional societies. Dr. Spencer is the author of numerous publications on topics ranging from malaria, filariasis, and schistosomiasis to the use of community health care workers in the control of disease.

CONSULTANTS

Thomas Denny, M.Sc., is an Associate Professor of Pathology, Laboratory Medicine and Pediatrics and Director of the Center for Laboratory Investigation at the New Jersey Medical School. Mr. Denny is the principal investigator of a $6.2 million grant from NIAID to develop the AIDS Immunology Quality Assessment Program. The program will be responsible for monitoring performance and developing new immunologic laboratory assays for 85 to 100 NIH-supported AIDS laboratories throughout the United States. He has more than 20 years of cellular immunology experience related to studying host defense mechanisms in response to tumors and/or infectious diseases. He has served on numerous committees for the NIH-NIAID Division of AIDS over the last two decades as part of the HIV clinical trials program. In 1997, he received a NIH HIV Innovative Vaccine Grant award to study a new method of vaccine delivery. He holds an M.Sc. in molecular and biomedical immunology from the University of East London and completed a course of study in strategic management at the Wharton School, University of Pennsylvania in 1991. He has completed the Program for Advanced Training in Biomedical Research Management at Harvard School of Public Health. Mr. Denny has authored and coauthored more than 70 peer-reviewed papers. In 1991, Mr. Denny helped establish a small laboratory in the Republic of Kalmykia (former Soviet Union) to improve the care of children with HIV/AIDS. In the aftermath of September 11, Mr. Denny established a medical school study to comprehensively assess immunologic memory/responses in those (individuals more than 30 years old) who had previously received smallpox vaccinations. He has recently been called upon to help support NIH biodefense vaccine trials. Mr. Denny's policy interests include vaccine development, regulatory issues, clinical trials, women and infant HIV/AIDS, accessibility to care, and global public health. Mr. Denny previously served as a Robert Wood Johnson Policy Fellow with the National Academies.

Bjorg Palsdottir, M.P.A., is the Cofounder and Associate Director of the Center for Global Health at New York University School of Medicine, dedicated to shaping new interdisciplinary education and capacity development strategies for health and health-allied professionals. Prior to working for the Center Ms. Palsdottir worked for the International Rescue Committee a relief and development organization, first at their headquarters in New York, then as a regional information coordinator for East and Central Africa covering programs in Sudan, Somalia, Rwanda, Burundi, Tanzania, Kenya, and the Democratic Republic of Congo. Her consultancy work has included the development of a management training program taught in Uganda and an evaluation of the American International Health Alliance's emergency medical training programs in Ukraine, Russia, and Uzbekistan. Prior to her working for humanitarian organizations, she worked as a journalist for *The Economist* Intelligence Unit in New York as well as for the Palestine-Israel Journal in Jerusalem. Ms. Palsdottir has also studied and worked in France, Germany, Denmark, Norway, Switzerland, and her home country of Iceland. She holds a B.A. in economic journalism, and a master's in Public Administration and a certificate in Management Training and Organizational Development from New York University; she is also a graduate of the Coaches Training Institute in San Rafael, California.

Claire Panosian, M.D., D.T.M.H. (London) (Senior Consultant/Writer), is a Professor of Medicine/Infectious Diseases at the David Geffen School of Medicine at UCLA, a tropical medicine and infectious diseases clinician, and a medical journalist. She joined the UCLA faculty after attending Stanford University and Northwestern University School of Medicine and completing her postgraduate medical training at Northwestern Medical Center, Tufts–New England Medical Center, and the London School of Hygiene and Tropical Medicine. Over the past 20 years, she has frequently worked overseas as a medical educator and has pioneered several global health curricula in the UCLA School of Medicine, UCLA College of Letters and Science, and UCLA Graduate School of Education. Her second career as a journalist includes 6 years as a medical writer, reporter, and coanchor for national medical television; she has also authored many articles and columns for *Scientific American, Discover* magazine, and the *Los Angeles Times*. Dr. Panosian is currently a Councilor of the American Society of Tropical Medicine and Hygiene and a senior consultant/writer for the Institute of Medicine Board on Global Health where she previously coedited *Saving Lives, Buying Time: Economics of Malaria Drugs in an Age of Resistance* (The National Academies Press, 2004). Her other medical publications include original research articles as well as chapters, reviews and editorials on parasitic infections, diarrhea, tuberculosis, malaria, and immunization.

Kai Spratt, R.N., M.P.H., Ph.D., has more than 17 years of experience in the health care field. For the last 12 years she has been associated with Johns Hopkins University in a wide range of professional areas including: research, research design, strategic planning, monitoring, and evaluation, and project management. Dr. Spratt's HIV/AIDS expertise dates back to 1996 with her involvement on a HIVNET multidisciplinary team conducting HIV/AIDS epidemiological and behavioral surveillance and research in Pune, India, including Phase I trials assessing the efficacy of counseling methods and a vaginal microbicide. As a professional behavioral scientist, Dr. Spratt has made significant contributions to the design of HIV/AIDS and related projects in many countries in Asia, Africa, and Latin America. Seconded to the U.S. Agency for International Development from 1999–2001, Dr. Spratt served as the HIV/AIDS Technical Advisor to the Asia and Near East Bureau. In this capacity, Dr. Spratt conducted technical analyses; designed and developed strategic approaches to addressing HIV/AIDS; provided technical and programmatic guidance; developed monitoring and evaluation frameworks; and fostered key relationships for the Agency with government entities (both domestic and foreign), organizations working in the field of HIV/AIDS, and the international donor community. Dr. Spratt joined JHPIEGO in June 2001 as the Director of the Research and Evaluation Office and Senior HIV/AIDS Advisor. In January 2003 the Office of HIV/AIDS was opened under Dr. Spratt's direction, becoming the Center for Excellence in HIV/AIDS in July 2004; the Center provides technical assistance to JHPIEGO country programs and assures that best practices are disseminated throughout JHPIEGO programs. Dr. Spratt has technical expertise in the area of VCT, PMTCT, care and support, and monitoring and evaluation.

Richard Guerrant, M.D. (Liaison to the Board on Global Health), is the Thomas H. Hunter Professor of International Medicine in the Division of Infectious Diseases and International Health and Director of the Trans-University Center for Global Health at the University of Virginia School of Medicine. He received his M.D. at the University of Virginia with additional training in medicine and infectious diseases at Boston City Hospital, NIH, Johns Hopkins, and UVA. Dr. Guerrant has worked in the Congo, Bangladesh, and in a longstanding collaboration in Northeast Brazil and is past president of the American Society of Tropical Medicine. His primary areas of research include recognition, diagnosis, pathogenesis, and control of enteric infections; and in mentoring colleagues who return to develop Trans-University Centers for Global Health in Brazil, Ghana, Philippines, and South Africa. With colleagues in Brazil, Dr. Guerrant's research documents the effects of and potential solutions for diarrhea and enteric parasitic infections on the long-term physical and cognitive development in malnourished children and on anti-HIV drug absorption and resistance in patients with AIDS. Dr. Guerrant is the author of over 400 scientific and clinical articles and reviews. He also edits *At the Edge of Development: Health Crises in a Transitional Society*, and textbooks on *Infections in the GI Tract* and the two-volume textbook *Tropical Infectious Diseases: Principles, Pathogens and Practice*.

IOM STAFF

Patrick W. Kelley, M.D., Dr.P.H., joined the Institute of Medicine in July 2003 serving as the Director of the Board on Global Health and the Board on African Academy Science Development. Previously he served in the U.S. Army for more than 23 years as a physician, residency director, epidemiologist, and program manager. In his last DoD position, Dr. Kelley founded and directed the presidentially mandated DoD Global Emerging Infections Surveillance and Response System (DoD-GEIS). This responsibility entailed managing approximately $42 million dollars of emerging infections surveillance, response, training, and capacity-building activities undertaken in partnership numerous elements of the federal government and with health ministries in over 45 developing countries. He also designed and established the DoD Accessions Medical Standards Analysis and Research Activity, the first systematic DoD effort to apply epidemiology to the evidence-based development and evaluation of physical and psychological accession standards. Dr. Kelley is an experienced communicator having lectured in over 20 countries and authored over 50 scholarly papers and book chapters. He also designed and served as the specialty editor for the two-volume textbook *Military Preventive Medicine: Mobilization and Deployment.* Dr. Kelley obtained his M.D. from the University of Virginia and his Dr.P.H. from the Johns Hopkins School of Hygiene and Public Health.

Patricia Cuff, M.S., R.D., M.P.H., is currently the Study Director for the Committee on the Options for Overseas Placement of US Health Professionals. She was most recently a Study Director with the Board on Neuroscience and Behavioral Health. Ms. Cuff joined the Institute of Medicine staff in April, 2001, to work on the report, *Emerging Microbial Threats to Health in the 21st Century* with the Board on Global Health. Prior to that, she worked extensively in the field of HIV-nutrition as a counselor, researcher, and lecturer on topics of adult and pediatric HIV. She received an M.S. in nutrition and an M.P.H. in Population and Family Health from Columbia University in 1995, and performed her undergraduate studies at the University of Connecticut.

Alyson Schwaber joined the Institute of Medicine in November 2004 as a research associate for the Committee on the Options for Overseas Placement of U.S. Health Professionals. Prior to joining the National Academies, Ms. Schwaber was a program manager for sustainable development focused on Africa at Sister Cities International in Washington, D.C. She served as a Peace Corps community health volunteer in Mauritania from 1999– 2001. Following her service, she remained in Mauritania for two additional years to work with an international NGO on their newly created

HIV/AIDS project. Ms. Schwaber completed her undergraduate studies at Penn State University and is currently pursuing a Master of Public Health degree at Johns Hopkins University.

Dianne Stare is a Research Assistant for the Board on Global Health. Ms. Stare began her tenure with the National Academies in 2001 as a Project Assistant with the Board on Radiation Effects Research in the Division of Earth and Life Studies. There she worked on studies relating to compensation claims of radiation-exposed veterans, evaluating radioactive fallout exposure to the U.S. population, and several CDC studies related to the Hanford Nuclear Reservation. Ms. Stare joined the Board on Global Health in 2003 and is currently involved with the Committee on the Options for Overseas Placement of US Health Professionals and the InterAcademy Medical Panel Secretariat. Prior to joining the Academies, Ms. Stare managed a clinical drug study in Buenos Aires, Argentina, and coordinated laboratory research for the Penn State Cancer Center. Ms. Stare received her B.S. in Biology from Syracuse University.

Allison L. Berger is a Senior Program Assistant for the Board on Global Health. She currently provides meeting and travel assistance on an Institute of Medicine fast-track study "Committee on the Options for Overseas Placement of U.S. Health Professionals." Ms. Berger previously served as a Project Assistant for the IOM's Medical Follow-up Agency, and the Board on Neuroscience and Behavioral Health where she worked on other IOM studies: *Noise-Induced Hearing Loss and Tinnitus in the Military; Health Literacy: A Prescription to End Confusion*; and *Introducing Behavioral and Social Science into Medical School Curricula*. Before joining the IOM staff, she served a 5-year tenure as an Administrative Assistant for the American Psychological Association where she assisted the APA Committee on Psychological Test and Assessment, Committee on Scientific Awards, and the Committee on Animal Research and Ethics. She also worked on several funding and grant programs sponsored by the APA Science Directorate.